An Electronic Silent Spring

Facing the Dangers and Creating Safe Limits

Katie Singer

Portal Books | 2014

2014
Portal Books | Distributed by SteinerBooks
610 Main St., Great Barrington, MA 01230
www.steinerbooks.org

Cover image and design by Kendra Arnold

Author photo by Jeremy Green

Publication of this work was made possible in part by a grants from the F&S Fund, Santa Fe Community Foundation; New Hampshire Charitable Foundation; and the Bloom-Frankel Family Fund, a donor advised fund of Combined Jewish Philanthropies of Greater Boston, Inc.

Author's Disclaimer

This material has been created solely for educational purposes. The author and publisher are not engaged in providing electrical or medical advice or services. The author and publisher provide this information and the reader accepts it with the understanding that everything done or tried as a result of reading this book is at his or her own risk. The author and publisher shall have neither liability nor responsibility to any person or entity with respect to any loss, damage, or injury caused or alleged to be caused directly or indirectly by the information contained in this book.

Library of Congress Cataloging-in-Publication Data

Singer, Katie, 1960–
An electronic silent spring : facing the dangers and creating safe limits / Katie Singer.
pages cm
Includes bibliographical references and index.
ISBN 978-1-938685-10-1 (hardcover)—ISBN 978-1-938685-08-8 (pbk.)—ISBN 978-1-938685-09-5 (ebook)
1. Electromagnetic waves—Health aspects. 2. Stray currents—Physiological effect. I. Title. II. Title: Silent spring.
QP82.2.E43S56 2014
612'.014481—dc23

2014006010

An Electronic Silent Spring

Issues Covered in this Book

While they operate, mobile phones, mobile phone chargers, iPads, cellular antennas, Wi-Fi, compact fluorescent lights, transformers, and "smart" utility meters emit electromagnetic radiation (EMR) at frequencies and amplitudes that are not found in nature. *An Electronic Silent Spring* describes how wildlife and peoples' health are affected.

1. The book reports on peer-reviewed studies that show that EMR-exposed tadpoles die, aspen tree seedlings wither, bee colonies collapse, birds crash into antennas, and white stork mates fight.
2. Signals emitted by metal detectors, "smart" utility meters, hybrid cars, and other common electronics can shut off a medical implant. While the FDA regulates microwave ovens (whose signals can interfere with cardiac pacemakers), no agency regulates cell phones, which operate closer to the body, with more power and at the same frequency as a microwave oven. Geophysicist, electrical engineer, and implant patient Dr. Gary Olhoeft explains the issues.
3. Dr. Martha Herbert, Harvard pediatric neurologist, and Cindy Sage, MA, coeditor of the BioInitiative Report, and others explain why exposing children to Wi-Fi may lead to autism. The American Academy of Pediatrics warns pregnant women and children not to use cell phones.
4. Federal regulations protect the engineering needs of electronic devices and telecom companies. Federal law prohibits local officials from refusing installation of a cell tower based on health or environmental concerns. The book explains federal policies, which do not recognize that EMR can harm health.
5. Underwriters Lloyds of London and A.M. Best advise companies not to insure against damages to health caused by wireless devices. This book presents the peer-reviewed studies underlying analysts' concerns.

Katie Singer's *An Electronic Silent Spring* also offers an extensive solutions section for policy makers, telecom and utility companies, schools, civic groups, and individuals who want to reduce EMR emissions and exposure.

DEDICATED TO THIS BOOK'S CONTRIBUTORS,

WHOSE LOVE FOR THE EARTH AND HUMANITY

MAKES THESE PAGES SING

Author's Notes

To protect peoples' privacy, I have sometimes changed identifying characteristics.

Throughout this book, I refer to digital, wireless, transmitting utility meters as "smart" meters. The industry has trademarked the term SmartMeters. When reprinting letters by others who have written about these meters, I have kept the spelling true to their original letters.

Used by Permission

Letter from the American Academy of Pediatrics to Representative Dennis Kucinich.

Letter from De-Kun Li, MD, PhD, MPH to the California Council on Science and Technology.

"My Life Six Feet Under Ten Cell Antennas" by Veronica Ciandre.

Excerpt from *Bees, Birds and Mankind* by Warner Ulrich.

Please check www.electronicsilentspring.com for updates to this book.

The consequences of undervaluing or misjudging the biological effects of long-term, low-level exposure (to electromagnetic radiation emanating from radar, television, communications systems, microwave ovens, industrial heat-treatment systems, and many other sources) could become a critical problem for the public health, especially if genetic effects are involved.

from "Program for Control of Electromagnetic Pollution of the Environment," authored by The Electromagnetic Radiation Management Advisory Council, issued by The President's Office of Telecommunications Policy, in 1971

CONTENTS

Introduction

Given that humans have existed for well over 150,000 years, electrical and wireless technologies are *very* recent developments. We became able to generate and manipulate electricity only two hundred years ago. Yet our global economic, medical, educational, utility, military and other systems now depend on digital electronics. Most people who are alive now cannot imagine life without them or a mobile phone.

Electricity, electronics, and wireless devices have created profound benefits for humanity. They have also created hazards for our health and for wildlife.

Consider this book a forum that introduces vocabulary, personal experiences, scientific studies, questions, and solutions about electrosmog. Consider me a student of things electric—and the forum's moderator. While physicists, biologists, doctors, engineers, lawyers, and citizens may speak apparently different languages—and rarely with each other, we begin to communicate here. People who give testimony may disagree with each other or give conflicting reports. Sometimes, information is simplified in a way that renders it slightly inaccurate.

I have aimed to encourage discussion about what we can and cannot control around electrical issues. As you read, please write down your questions—and research them. We need many researchers and many forums. May every person be recognized as the expert in their experience. May we all recognize that every action affects the whole.

My sincere thanks to every person who joins this roundtable.

About the book's title: Before the marine biologist Rachel Carson published *Silent Spring* in 1962, few people understood the consequences of spraying a backyard, a farm, or recreational park with pesticides. Her book inspired the creation of the Environmental Protection Agency (EPA) and led to generations of environmental activism.

We all stand on the shoulders of Rachel Carson. May this book's title serve to attract the attention that its issues deserve.

In the stories that follow, some names and identifying characteristics have been changed to protect peoples' privacy.

Katie Singer
February 2014

I

Give Me a Megaphone

Please note that throughout this book, personal stories and scientists' testimonies are presented in italics—unless, as with this story from Ginger Farver, the entire chapter is in one person's voice.

For his first twenty-five years, my son Rich was healthy. He was six feet, two inches tall and two hundred pounds. He kept fit by playing basketball and riding his bike just about everywhere. Since he was a Democrat and I was a Republican, we had a lot of debates. Usually, he won.

In the fall of 2005, Rich started working on a master's degree in political science at San Diego State University. During his first few months at SDSU, he called me every day from his cell phone, crying. "Mom, just stay on with me," he'd say. And of course, I did. I knew something was off, but I didn't know what to do about it. He'd never had panic attacks before.

Soon enough, Rich fell in love with the school and with San Diego. He worked as a teaching assistant and spent seven days a week in Room 131 of Nasatir Hall, the political science building. He wrote his master's thesis on the politics of stadium building. In his graduation picture, in the Spring of 2006, he squinted. One of his eyes would not open all the way.

Rich stayed in San Diego and applied for law school. He told me that even if he got in, he wasn't sure if he should attend, because he'd developed short-term memory problems.

In the Fall of 2007, Craig, my husband, and I went to visit our son. We'd pick him up in the morning and run errands. Then Rich would go back to his apartment for a nap until dinner time.

We didn't get it.

Rich's girlfriend told us, "He gets headaches a lot. He curls up like a cat and sleeps by the patio window—every day."

Before leaving, I noticed a vein on the right side of Rich's hairline that traveled to his right eye, just above his eyebrow. A few months later, he developed problems with his balance, and he had nosebleeds every morning. We thought it was a deviated septum, which I'd had. He scheduled a doctor's appointment for March 14, 2008.

Thursday evening, March 13, I was home checking email. Craig was taking a shower. The phone rang, and Rich whispered, "Mom?" He had the worst headache of his life, and he'd been projectile vomiting all over his apartment.

"Get an ambulance immediately," I told him. *"Get to the hospital."*

The emergency room doctor called us at one in the morning. Rich had bleeding on the brain. He'd had a seizure and would need more testing.

Craig and I took out our suitcases. I was so disoriented that I only packed underwear. At the airport, we told the attendant, "We don't care what it costs, get us to San Diego."

Ten days later, Rich, Craig and I sat in the neurosurgeon's office. The doctor said, "glioblastoma multiforme brain cancer."

Everyone knows what a brain cancer diagnosis means. The life we'd known until then was over. I kept myself together so I could be there for Rich and talk with the doctor. I could not pronounce glioblastoma multiforme, but I could ask, "What causes it?"

The doctor replied, "Using a cell phone."

Why had I never heard this before? I wrapped an arm around myself. None of us had a landline anymore. My cell phone was in my purse. Rich's and Craig's were parked in their pockets.

We took our son to the Tisch Brain Tumor Center at Duke University. Ted Kennedy was released the day we arrived. I figured if Tisch was the best place for Senator Kennedy, then it was the best place for Rich. We did everything for him that we could come up with, and still, he had blackouts and went blind. His cancer didn't go away.

Another one of his doctors told me, "Your son's tumor isn't caused by genetics." I wrote his words in a journal like a clue I might understand later.

Before Rich came home, we got rid of our cell phones and cordless phones. We used only corded landlines to minimize our exposure to radiation. We quit our Wi-Fi and got cabled Internet access.

For Rich's last month, Craig took off from work, and Lee, our elder son, moved back in. Rich didn't want to use a walker or a cane to get from one room to the next, even though he was so wobbly. I'm only 5' 3", so I couldn't help him. Craig and Lee had to do it.

Rich died October 11, 2008, seven months after his seizure.

For a long time, I just stayed in bed. I was so numb that I felt lucky to make it to the couch.

After a few months, I got curious about glioblastoma multiforme (GBM) and cell phones. I started doing research. At first, I had to look up each word so I could make sense of it. But now I can explain it. And that is what I want to do. Because Rich would want his colleagues and friends to know what I have learned. And because I do not want any other parent to go through what Craig and I have gone through.

From 2001, when he was twenty-two, until his seizure in 2008, Rich used a cell phone every day for two to three hours. So he had a wireless device emitting radiation beside his brain all that time. A study in Sweden found that for every one hundred hours of cell phone use, the risk of brain cancer increases by 5%.[1] For every year of cell phone use, the risk of brain cancer increases by 8%.[2] With two to three thousand cumulative hours of analog cell phone use, there is a 490% increased risk of brain cancer.[3] (Rich used an analog cell phone. Current mobile phones are digital, not analog. Digital phones emit more radiation than the kind used in these studies.)

There's a barrier around the brain that keeps toxins in the blood from entering the brain. Using a cell phone for two hours weakens this barrier. A leak in the barrier can contribute to a brain tumor.

Nine months after Rich died, I found an article online about a suspected cancer cluster at San Diego State University. Four people who all spent time in Nasatir Hall's room 131 had gotten brain cancer. Room 131 was a lounge and an office for people who worked in SDSU's political science department. One of Rich's professors told me that he practically lived in that room. The article reported that there are cellular antennas on the Communications building beside Nasatir Hall. Three of the people, including a graduate student, had died.

That was my son.

---

1 Mild et al, "Pooled analysis of two Swedish case-control studies on the use of mobile and cordless telephones and the risk of brain tumours diagnosed during 1997–2003, *International Journal of Occupational Safety and Ergonomics*, (JOSE) 13 (1) (2007) 63-71.3.

2 Ibid.

3 Hardell et al, "Pooled analysis of two case-control studies on use of cellular and cordless telephones and the risk for malignant brain tumors diagnosed in 1997–2003. *International Archives of Occupational and Environmental Health*, 79; 9-8-2006, 630–639.

I read the article about twenty times, and then I ended up on the floor.

I started doing research about the cell tower beside Nasatir Hall where Rich spent so much time. It's a GWEN tower, installed at the highest point on campus. GWEN stands for Ground Wave Emergency Network. The antennas' signals are used for police, ambulance and Homeland Security networks. They're needed for cell phones and WiMax. SDSU's antennas were upgraded in the summer of 2005, around the time Rich arrived. Their signals broadcast for seventy-two miles and can penetrate most structures.

GWEN towers are common on campuses across the country.

The tower also holds "cell dishes" that are part of the High Performance Wireless Research and Educational Network (HPWREN) project. These dishes provide Internet connections for SDSU, the Mount Palomar Observatory, and for Native American land. They also link CalFire and other agencies to the Internet during emergencies.

If an antenna's signals can penetrate most structures, wouldn't they also penetrate people? I could not imagine that hanging out under a tower of powerful antennas is safe, so I wrote SDSU's administration.

They replied that "the equipment is FCC (Federal Communications Commission) approved and does not include any unusual signal strength."

What happens when you use a cell phone for two hours a day *and* you hang out in a building that's beside a cell tower?

I contacted SDSU's president, Stephen Weber, and its Board of Directors and requested a toxicology study of Nasatir Hall. The University hired Thomas Mack, an epidemiologist, to study the situation and write a report. His third paragraph states, "I have not been informed of any unusual chemical or radiation exposure to persons working in this building, and I therefore presume there are none."

I realized that SDSU considers Dr. Mack's report the end of the matter, so I contacted Governor Schwarzenegger. He said it sounded like a campus issue and referred me back to the campus.

I made a list of people who spent time in Nasatir Hall near this antenna and who got cancer:

Employee #1 died in 1993 of a GBM brain tumor. There was an antenna on SDSU then, which sent signals from radio and TV studios to transmitters on Mount Miguel. It was removed from SDSU in 1995.

Employee #2 was diagnosed with brain cancer and died in 2008.

Employee #3 was diagnosed with brain cancer in 2008.

Employee #4 also died of some kind of cancer in 2008.

Rich Farver, 29, was diagnosed with GBM in March, 2008; he died in October, 2008.

This list raised a lot of questions for me. I decided I needed to visit San Diego State again. I called a hotel and got to talking with the man who answered the phone. His friend works at SDSU, and got diagnosed with a GBM brain tumor in 2008. This woman does not use a cell phone very much. But the building where she works also has GWEN and HPWREN antennas. I put her on my list, *Employee #5*.

Craig and I drove back to SDSU a year after Rich died, in the Fall of 2009. Room 131 in Nasatir Hall was closed, presumably because it needs renovation. Now, students hang out in the court underneath the cell tower. I watched them laugh with their professors. I watched them sleep, study, talk on mobile phones and use their laptops right under the tower.

I wanted a megaphone. I wanted to tell every single one of them to get clear of this place.

I know these towers are on other schools. If any mother thinks her kids are safe, she is sadly mistaken.

In August 2010, *SDSU Employee #6*, who worked in a building near a GWEN tower, died of brain cancer.

In March, 2011, a video was posted on YouTube about an SDSU student with brain cancer. This student may have been diagnosed before arriving at SDSU. *Student #2*.

In the Spring of 2012, an undergraduate who lived on campus across the street from a GWEN tower and who took classes in a building near another GWEN tower died of undisclosed causes while taking a nap. *Student #3*.

In January, 2013, *Employee #7*, who worked in Nasatir Hall under a GWEN tower died of some form of cancer.

After we learned about all the harm that comes from cigarettes and put warnings on their packages, I figured that whatever I buy has been tested and determined to be safe by a government agency and by the company that sells it.

I know now that this is naive thinking.

Now, I don't mince words. I tell people that using a mobile phone increases your risk of brain cancer. If you think that increasing your risk is your personal business, that may be true. But since every mobile phone requires antennas, then your choice to use a wireless device exposes the rest of us to radiation—with no choice in the matter at all.

Smartphones are even more dangerous than the kind Rich used, because they can transmit more data—and so they need more bandwidth. Their antennas emit more radiation. If you don't want an antenna in your neighborhood, quit your mobile phone.

A friend, who's a teacher, asked me to speak to her class when they studied the causes of cancer. I told these ten-year-olds what happened to Rich, and one boy shared that his father died from a brain tumor. For me, the worst part was that this child has a cell phone. "Please," I begged him. "For my sake, throw that phone away."

A girl asked, "At what age is it okay to have a cell phone?"

"If you were my child," I told her, "it would never be okay."

Also recently, two of Rich's childhood friends were diagnosed with GBM brain tumors. One of them had a seizure while driving. Fortunately, an alert passenger took the wheel, and no accident occurred.

In my grief support group, there's a couple whose daughter was bicycling around her neighborhood a month after Rich died. A woman talking on her cell phone drove into this girl and killed her.

Everywhere I turn, it seems, the risks of using this technology far outweigh what anyone could get from it.

I will never have a cell phone again, and my life is much simpler. I engage in actual conversation now. If I go out of town and need to borrow a landline, most folks are courteous. For emergencies, we could have phone booths along the highways, just like the good old days.

Because of Rich, I've learned a lot about public policy. I've learned that we need to keep landlines and corded phones. We need laws that protect our environment and peoples' health from radiation emitted by wireless devices, cellular antennas and "smart" utility meters. In the U.S., epidemiologists need access to cell phone use records so that they can determine the health effects of using mobile phones and living near antennas—just like researchers in Sweden are allowed. Every person needs proper warnings about the dangers of mobile devices and transmitting antennas. The Cell Phone Right to Know Act would get us started on these regulations.

I like to think that Rich would be pleased with me, for how much I have learned—and for voicing it. I like to think he did not die in vain.

2

My Life Six Feet Under Ten Cell Antennas

by Veronica Ciandre

In November, 2009, an array of cell phone antennas was placed on Veronica Ciandre's apartment building in downtown Toronto. Like the building's other residents, she learned about the installation as the cranes arrived. Ms. Ciandre first posted this story at magdahavas.com in 2010.

If you had told me three months ago not to hold a cell phone to my head or body, I would have listened politely. But I wouldn't have changed a thing.

If you had told me to exchange my cordless phones for old-fashioned corded phones, I would have listened. But I wouldn't have changed anything. I *liked* my cordless phones.

If you had told me to use an Ethernet cable with my laptop and to keep Airplane mode turned on, or to move the Wi-Fi router from my bedroom and to turn it off at night and when not in use, or to get rid of my Wi-Fi altogether, I would have wondered, *why* would I want to do any of that?

If you had told me three months ago that baby monitors should not be placed near babies, or to ask my fourteen-year-old daughter to text more than talk and not to sleep with her phone or computer on the pillow beside her, or to replace every fluorescent lightbulb with an incandescent one, I would have listened. But I probably would not have changed a thing.

If you had told me that the microwave radiation emitted by cell phones, cordless phones, Wi-Fi, cellular antennas, and other wireless technologies causes people to experience all manner of symptoms from insomnia to high blood pressure and heart palpitations and anxiety and should be avoided completely or at least whenever possible, I still wouldn't have changed a thing. After all, the government approves of these devices, and the media tell us that they're safe.

But before three months ago, I had not lived six feet under ten cellular antennas that were installed on the roof above my balcony. Before three months ago, I had health and vitality. I slept like a baby. I did not wake up with numb hands and feet, my body feeling prickly all night and tingling or vibrating almost all day. I did not spend night after night in a hyperactive state feeling like electricity was running through me.

Before, I lived in a home that I loved. It was my sanctuary. I did not have hissing, buzzing, or high-pitched ringing in my ear. I did not ever get tension headaches. I did not feel an invisible band wrapped around my head creating pressure. I did not feel bouts of nausea on a regular basis, sometimes accompanied by a metallic taste in my mouth, and I did not get dizzy spells.

I was not afraid that I might have a heart attack as I slept on a makeshift floor mattress in my living room and felt my heart race all night. I was not without focus or direction or ability to concentrate. I had never felt shocks from touching my mattress, my light switches, my pots or my cats.

My daughter did not have inexplicable rashes that hurt "in" her skin (as she described it). She did not have headaches or feel nauseous and dizzy in our home or experience the blood in her hand going cold. She never had sleepless nights.

Before three months ago, I had not talked with someone who could have sold me thousands of dollars worth of products by convincing me that they would alleviate the situation, but advised me, instead, "If you care about your health and your daughter, get out of there. You have to move."

I had never abandoned my home. I had never couch-surfed with my fourteen-year-old in tow while trying to maintain some semblance of a normal life. I had not spent fifteen days getting two hours of sleep each night because my body vibrated all the time. I had not cried for hours feeling like I was losing my mind from sleep deprivation and from feeling fight-or-flight twenty-four hours each day.

I had not researched everything I could find to educate myself about the dangers of exposure to human-made electromagnetic frequencies and microwave radiation. I was not fully aware of cellular antennas and the invisible wireless web that continues to grow around all of our heads.

I could not tell the difference between a Bell cell antenna, a Rogers, Globealive, Tellus, or Wind cell antenna. I had never heard of Industry Canada or Spectrum, Canada Safety Code 6 or the *BioInitiative Report.*

I had not spoken to Health Canada, Industry Canada, the Canadian Environmental Legal Association, Environmental Health Clinic, Environmental Health Association, the Environmental Protection Office, the Toronto Environmental Alliance, Canadian Association of Physicians for the Environment, or my city councilors' office, trying to find out whether it's safe to live six feet under ten cellular antennas. So far, none of them have told me, "It's not safe." But thankfully, I have a body that tells me the truth, and the good judgment to listen to my body.

Before three months ago, I did not have clear and unpleasant physical reactions to my cell phone or the cell phones used by people near me. I did not get off of busses because half of the passengers were texting or talking and the RF signals bouncing around the bus were more than my body could handle. I did not react to the touch of my computer keyboard or from sitting close to the monitor for too long. I did not feel my legs tingling and going slightly numb if I spent too much time in a room with Wi-Fi. I didn't feel nauseous and have sharp pains go through my hand and up my arm if I made a call with a cordless phone or a cell phone. I did not feel nauseous if I sat for too long or too close to a television.

I do for now.

Before three months ago, I could not have told you when I stood within four blocks of a cellular antenna installation. I never thought twice about leaning on walls or in close proximity to the electrical wiring in a room, or lying on the floor above a basement for the same reasons. I never considered the effects of my neighbors' Wi-Fi and cordless phone base stations broadcasting through the walls between us.

I had not heard the words "electrosensitive" or "electrohypersensitive." I had not spent hours and hours on the phone trying to find a doctor who knows what a cellular antenna is and the effects of living six feet under ten of them. The few I found who knew what I was talking about and who offer treatment that would have been good for me cost an arm or a leg and a plane ticket.

Before three months ago, I had not stayed in six places over nine days just trying to get a good night's sleep. Because even after friends and family unplugged their Wi-Fi and cordless phones and everything but the fridge, my body reacted to their neighbors' wireless devices, which emitted through the walls to where I tried to sleep.

Before, I only knew the benefits of wireless devices. I had not heard of EMF Solutions, Earthcalm, magdahavas.com, the WEEP Initiative, the Electrosensitive Society, safelivingtechnologies.com, a Q-link, a gauss meter or an electro-smog meter. I had not read stories from hundreds of people around the world whose lives have been profoundly impacted by something we have come to believe is purely beneficial and harmless, something we cannot see: microwave radiation from wireless devices that emit at levels not meant for human absorption.

Three months ago, I was blindsided. My life got turned upside down by radiation from cellular antennas. Now, I'm looking for a new home. I'm challenged by the fact that I've got to consider my recently acquired "sensitivities" more than the home's location, size, cost, or style.

Please, pay attention. Pay attention to the choices you make and the ones that others make for you. Pay attention now, before you pay dearly.

3

Wildlife Health and Radio-Frequency Fields

The radio-frequency (RF) signals that cellular antennas, mobile devices and "smart" utility meters require to function are now ubiquitously and continuously emitted.

How do these signals affect wildlife?

Scientists report that RF fields emitted by cellular antennas alone potentially cause the decline of animal populations, reduction of some species' useful territory, and deterioration of plant health. Some species may experience reduction of their natural defenses, problems in reproduction, and aversive behavioral responses.[1]

Here are summaries of studies about the effects of RF signals on trees, insects, frogs, and birds:

Trees

In a 2010 paper published in the *International Journal of Forestry Research*, researcher Katie Haggerty explained that the Earth's natural radio frequency environment has remained about the same within the lifespan of modern trees. "Before 1800," Haggerty wrote, "the major components of this environment were broadband radio noise from space (galactic noise), from

1 A. Balmori, Electromagnetic pollution from phone masts. Effects on wildlife," *Pathophysiology*, (2009), doi; 10.1016/j.pathophys.2009.01.007.

lightning (atmospheric noise), and a smaller RF component from the sun.[2] ... Plants may have evolved" to use these environmental signals, along with visible light to regulate their periodic functions. Therefore, they may be sensitive to human-made RF fields. "The background of RF pollution," Haggerty continued, "is now many times stronger than the naturally occurring RF environment. From the perspective of evolutionary time, the change can be considered sudden and dramatic.[3] Growth rates of plants [4] and fungi[5] can be increased or decreased by RF exposure. Exposure to RF signals can induce plants to produce more meristems, [6] affect root cell structure,[7] and induce stress response ... causing biochemical changes."[8]

Ms. Haggerty went on to describe her study of the influence of RF signals on trembling aspen seedlings. Seedlings

---

2 N. M. Maslin, "*HF Communications: A Systems Approach*," New York: Plenum Press, 1987.

3 Ibid.; E. H. Sanders et al, "Broadband spectrum survey at Los Angeles, California," NTIA Report 47–336, 1997.

4 I. Y. Petrov et al, "Possibility of correction of vital processes in plant cell with microwave radiation," in *Proceedings of IEEE International Symposium on Electromagnetic Compatibility*, pp. 234–235, Dec., 1991.

5 A. Berg and H. Berg, "Influence of ELF sinusoidal electromagnetic fields on proliferation and metabolic yield of fungi," *Electromagnetic Biology and Medicine*, v. 25, no. 1 (2006): 71–77.

6 M. Tafforeau et al, "Plant sensitivity to low intensity105 GHz electromagnetic radiation," *Bioelectromagnetics*, v. 25, no. 6 (2004): 403–407.

7 M. B. Bitonti et al, "Magnetic field affects meristem cell activity and cell differentiation in Zea mays roots," *Plant Biosystems*, v. 140, no. 1, 87–93, 2006; Wawrecki, W. et al, "Influence of a weak DC electric field on root meristem architecture," *Annals of Botany*, v. 100, no. 4 (2007): 791–796.

8 D. Roux et al, "Electromagnetic Fields (900 MHz) evoke consistent molecular responses in tomato plants," *Physiologia Plantarum*, v. 128, no. 2 (2006): 283–288.

that were shielded in a Faraday cage (a metal container that prevents RF radiation from entering) thrived. Seedlings that were exposed to RF signals showed necrotic lesions and abnormal coloring in their leaves.[9]

According to British biologist Dr. Andrew Goldsworthy, "Trees are now dying mysteriously from a variety of diseases in urban areas all over Europe. They also show abnormal photoperiodic responses. Many have cancer-like growths under the bark (phloem nodules). The bark may also split so that the underlying tissues become infected. All of these can be explained as a result of exposure to weak RF fields from mobile phones, their base stations, Wi-Fi and similar sources of weak non-ionizing radiation."[10]

Other scientists have found that trees in areas with high Wi-Fi activity suffer from bleeding fissures in their bark, the death of parts of leaves, and abnormal growth. In 2010, in the Netherlands, 70% of urban ash trees suffered from radiation sickness, including a "lead-like shine" on their leaves, indicating the leaves' oncoming death. In 2005, only 10% of ash trees suffered radiation sickness.[11]

Ants

Perhaps the first study to demonstrate that insects have an electrical sense came out in 1992. Biologist William MacKay and his colleagues showed that several kinds of ants were attracted

---

9 Katie Haggerty, "Adverse influence of radio frequency background on trembling aspen seedlings: Preliminary observations," *International Journal of Forestry Research*, 2010.

10 See www.mastsanity.org/health/research/299-why-our-urban-trees-are-dying-by-andrew-goldsworthy-2011.html.

11 See www.popsci.com/technology/article/2010-11/wi-fi-radiation-killing-trees.

to electrical fields. Indeed, ants can damage equipment that produces “attractive” electrical fields.[12]

In 2013, Belgian biologist Marie-Claire Cammaerts and Swedish neuroscientist Olle Johansson exposed ants to common wireless devices. The scientists placed a mobile phone under a tray, then placed ants on the tray. When the phone was off or on standby mode, the ants’ angular speed increased. Within two to three seconds of the scientists’ turning the phone on (able to receive or send calls), the ants’ angular speed increased and their linear speed decreased.

Exposed to a smartphone, the linear speed of “fresh” ants decreased; their angular speed increased. The ants’ speed changed similarly but more strongly when exposed to a DECT (cordless landline) phone. They had difficulty moving their legs and did not move toward their nest or their food site as usual. The ants were exposed to each of these two phones for three minutes, and took two to four hours to resume their normal behavior.

When Cammaerts and Johansson put a mobile phone on standby mode under the ants’ nest, the ants left their nest immediately, taking their eggs, larvae, and nymphs with them. They relocated far from the phone. Once the phone was removed, the ants returned to their original location.

After thirty minutes of exposure to a Wi-Fi router, the ants’ speed changed again, as did their foraging behavior. It took them six to eight hours to resume normal foraging. Several ants never recovered and were found dead a few days later.

When the scientists placed an ACER Aspire 2920 about twenty-five centimeters away, the insects appeared disturbed as soon as the computer was switched on. When the PC was

12 William MacKay et al, “Attraction of Ants (Hymenoptera: Formicidae) to Electric Fields,” *Journal of the Kansas Entomological Society*, v. 65, no. 1 (1992): 39–43.

switched on with its Wi-Fi function deactivated, the ants appeared undisturbed.

The researchers concluded that ants can be used as bio-indicators to reveal the biological effects of RF signals from some wireless devices. They also advised users to de-activate the Wi-Fi function of their PCs.[13]

Bees

Bees also have an electrical sense. Bees are positively charged, and flowers are negatively charged. These charges help pollen stick to bees' hair while they pollenate. In 2012, biologist Dominic Clarke and his colleagues showed that bees use their electrical sense to determine whether or not a flower has recently been visited by another bee—and is therefore worth visiting.[14,15]

In *Bees, Birds and Mankind: Effects of Wireless Communication Technologies* (Kentum, 2009), German scientist Ulrich Warnke states, "Bees and other insects, just as birds, use the Earth's magnetic field and high frequency electromagnetic energy such as light. They accomplish orientation and navigation by means of free radicals as well as a simultaneously reacting magnetite conglomerate. Technically produced electromagnetic oscillations in the MHz range and magnetic impulses in the low frequency range persistently disturb the natural orientation and navigation mechanisms created by evolution."

---

13 Marie-Claire Cammaerts and Olle Johansson, "Ants can be used as bio-indicators to reveal biological effects of electromagnetic waves from some wireless apparatus," *Electromagnetic Biology and Medicine*, 8.30.13.

14 Dominic Clarke et al, "Detection and learning of floral electric fields by bumblebees," *Science DOI*: 10.1126 /science.1230883; published online Feb. 21, 2013.

15 Matt Kaplan, "Bumblebees sense electric fields in flowers," *Nature*, Feb. 21, 2013.

In his book, Warnke quotes Ferdinand Ruzicka, a scientist and beekeeper who reported, in 2003, after several transmitters (cellular antennas) were erected in the immediate vicinity of his hives: "I observed a pronounced restlessness in my bee colonies (initially about forty) and a greatly increased urge to swarm. As a frame-hive beekeeper, I use a so-called high floor. The bees did not build their combs in the manner prescribed by the frames, but in random fashion. In the summer, bee colonies collapsed without obvious cause. In the winter, I observed that the bees went foraging despite snow and temperatures below zero, and they died of cold next to the hive. Colonies that exhibited this behavior collapsed, even though they were strong, healthy colonies with active queens before winter. They were provided with adequate additional food and the available pollen was more than adequate in autumn."

Ruzicka then organized a survey of beekeepers through the magazine *Der Bienen Vater.* All twenty of the beekeepers who replied to his questionnaire had a transmitter within 300 meters of their beehives. Compared to the bees' behavior before and after the transmitters were in operation, 37.5% observed increased aggression from their bees; 25% found that their bees had a greater tendency to swarm; 65% reported that their colonies were inexplicably collapsing since the transmitters became operational.

Warnke says that monocultures, pesticides, the Varroa mite, migratory beekeeping, dressed seed, severe winters, and genetically modified seeds could also explain the bee colonies' collapse. However, none of these convincingly explains "the fairly sudden and country-spanning appearance two to three years ago of the dying bees phenomenon. Should the bees simply be too weak or ill, they should also die in or near the hive. But no ill bees were found in research into this phenomenon."

In May, 2009, The U.S. Fish and Wildlife Service urged Congress to investigate the potential relationship between wireless devices and bee colony collapse.[16]

Frogs

In 2010, Spanish biologist Alfonso Balmori published his study of a common frog habitat 140 meters from a cellular antenna. The experiment lasted two months, from the egg phase until an advanced phase of tadpole. Balmori placed some of the frogs inside a Faraday cage. These shielded frogs had a mortality of 4.2%. The unshielded frogs—exposed to the antennas' RF fields—had a mortality of 90%. Balmori concluded that "this research may have huge implications for the natural world, which is now exposed to high microwave radiation levels from a multitude of phone masts."[17]

Bird collisions with telecom equipment

Albert Manville, PhD, wildlife biologist with the Division of Migratory Bird Management, U.S. Fish and Wildlife Service (USFWS), estimates that up to 6.8 million birds die per year in collisions with communications antennas or their guy-support wires in North America. The impacts of cellular antenna radiation on migratory birds in North America, especially those nesting close to these structures, remain suspect and unknown.

❈

Dr. Manville, January 2012: *Recent studies from Europe raise troubling concerns about the effects of radiation from cellular communication antennas, especially on resident, breeding*

16 See http://electromagnetichealth.org/electromagnetichealth-blog/emf-and-warnke-report-on-bees-birds-and-mankind/.

17 A. Balmori and C. Navarra, "Mobile phone mast effects on common frog (*Rana temporaria*) tadpoles; the city turned into a laboratory," *Electromagnetic Biology and Medicine*, v. 29 no. 1–2 (2010): 31–5, 59.

migratory birds. These apparent effects include feather deformities, weight loss, weakness, reduced survivorship and death, especially to those birds and their offspring nesting adjacent to cellular antennas. Where Before–After, Control-Impact (BACI) studies were performed during some of the European research, no effects to resident birds were detected prior to construction and operation of cellular communication antennas. Some laboratory studies in the U.S. have documented lethal effects of extremely low levels of radiation to chicken embryos in the frequencies of cellular telephones,[18] but research to better address cause and effect to wild birds in North America has yet to be conducted. To date, only anecdotal reports from instances in North America have been brought to the attention of authorities at the USFWS.

If we are to better understand the cumulative effects of human infrastructure on migratory birds—including communication technologies, research needs to be conducted to specifically address how radiation is affecting migratory birds and what resultant lethal and injurious effects are occurring. The explosive growth of hand-held technologies raises further concerns since potential impacts may grow.

The unpermitted killing or injury of a migratory bird, is called a "take" under the Migratory Bird Treaty Act (MBTA). The USFWS does not permit the 'incidental or accidental take' of any of the 1,007 migratory bird species protected under MBTA. Therefore, studies need to be undertaken to determine how much 'take' is occurring as a result of radiation, and what steps can be undertaken to "avoid or minimize" future "take." The USFWS continues to suggest to the FCC the need for these North American studies based alone on cumulative effects that must be addressed under National

18 A. Di Carlo. et al, "Chronic electromagnetic field exposure decreases HSP70 levels and lowers cytoprotection," *Journal of Cellular Biochemistry*, v. 84 (2002): 447–454.

Environmental Policy Act review. The studies need to better tease out how and at what level "takes" are occurring, then determine what conservation measures can be adopted to "avoid or minimize" future "take." Because of the controversial nature of this issue, any studies and outcomes need to be seamless and fully transparent.

The White Stork

During the Springs of 2002, 2003, and 2004, biologist Alfonso Balmori monitored the reproduction of the white stork, a vulnerable bird species that usually lives in urban areas. White stork couples build their nests in pinnacles and other very high places that are now exposed to human-made microwaves. Balmori studied white stork nests within 200 meters of antennas and nests located more than 300 meters from antennas. He found that 40% of the nests within 200 meters of antennas had no chicks, while only 3.3% of nests further than 300 meters of antennas had no chicks. Also, near antennas, white stork couples frequently fought for sticks, their sticks fell to the ground while they tried to build nests, the nests did not get built and hatched white stork chicks frequently died.[19]

Common citizens have also observed changes in birds when technologies that emit EMR are deployed. After transmitting water meters were installed in Renton, Washington in December 2012, a retired civil engineer who had spent thirty dollars per month on birdseed for years noticed that the feeders in his yard no longer emptied. His neighbors also noticed that immediately after the transmitting water meters were installed, the birds that had frequented their yard (beside a greenbelt) disappeared.[20]

19 A. Balmori, "Possible effects of electromagnetic fields from phone masts on a population of white stork (Ciconia ciconia)," *Electromagnetic Biology and Medicine,* v. 24 (2005): 109–119.

20 Brian Beckley, "Are 'smart' meters chasing away birds from Rolling Hills?" *Renton Reporter*, Feb. 22, 2013.

Birds, Bees and Magnetically-Sensitive Cryptochromes

Why would RF signals disturb birds and bees?

Andrew Goldsworthy, PhD, biologist: *To navigate and also to control their immune systems, birds and bees use magnetically-sensitive substances called cryptochromes. These are pigments found in virtually all animals, plants and many bacteria. Cryptochromes absorb blue-green and ultra-violet light and use this energy to drive photochemical reactions where light energy is converted to chemical energy. Cryptochromes measure light to control and reset animals' and plants' biological clocks. Some animals also use cryptochromes to sense the direction of the Earth's magnetic field.*

Unfortunately, cryptochromes are badly impaired by human-made oscillating fields that are orders of magnitude weaker than the Earth's steady magnetic field. Such impairment can disrupt insects' and animals' solar and magnetic navigational abilities. It can account for colony collapse disorder in bees, the loss of some migratory birds and butterflies, and immune system weakening in many more organisms.

An array of cryptochrome molecules oriented in different directions can be found in the compound eye of an insect, or in the retina of a vertebrate's eye. This cryptochrome found in the eyes is quite distinct from the regular visual pigments (rhodopsins) that are used in normal vision. However, the combination of these pigments gives the animal the potential to "see" the direction of the magnetic field, possibly as an extra color superimposed on its normal field of vision.

Robins can navigate in the Earth's magnetic field if they receive light from wavelengths absorbed by cryptochrome.[21] *However, exposure to human-made frequencies between 0.1 and 10MHz at field strengths as little as 0.085 mT (about 500*

21 T. Ritz et al, *Nature*, v. 429, 5-13-2004, 177–180.

times weaker than the Earth's magnetic field) made the birds completely unable to respond to the Earth's field.

Frequencies used by mobile devices, including cell phones, DECT cordless landline phones and Wi-Fi, can blot out "magnetic vision." Even lower field strengths are likely to disturb magnetic navigation, since radiation that is too weak to blot out magnetic vision totally may still be strong enough to distort a bird's perception of the Earth's field, causing the bird or insect to fly in the wrong direction.

The sheer number of wireless devices gives birds continuously conflicting navigational data—as if they're constantly bombarded by flashing disco lights. We should not be surprised that birds would leave such areas. Likewise, scientists who put DECT cordless phone base stations next to their beehives found that their bees behaved abnormally and were less likely to return to the hive.[22] *(Beekeepers are thereby well advised not to carry their mobile phones when visiting their hives.)*

Birds, bees and many other animals can also navigate by the sun's position. To do this, they must have an internal clock that adjusts to the sun's changing position throughout the day. Cryptochrome makes this clock sensitive to magnetic fields. A 300 mT steady field can alter the clock's speed or even stop it altogether.[23] *Given that sensing light and magnetic fields by cryptochrome uses the same basic mechanics as the internal clock, it's likely that weak alternating fields would also disrupt a clock's normal functions. As a consequence, weak, human-made electromagnetic fields would render animals unable to adjust accurately to the sun's changing position. This leaves the animal unable to use either magnetic or solar navigation. If there were no landmarks to guide it, the animal would be*

22 T. Yoshi et al, http://tinyurl.com/rans84.

23 T. Yoshi et al, http://tinyurl.com/cx7xaa.

completely lost. This could explain colony collapse disorder, when bees do not return to their hives.

Circadian (daily) metabolic rhythms, which occur in virtually all higher organisms, keep us in sync with the Earth's twenty-four hour rotation on its axis. Circadian rhythms are also driven by cryptochrome-containing internal clocks. They enable the organism to anticipate the coming of dawn and dusk, and they modify its metabolism to be ready for the new conditions. Circadian rhythms control the production of melatonin (a sleep hormone); at night, they divert metabolic resources to repair and immune system strengthening.

Losing or even weakening of the circadian rhythm—due to a failure of the internal clock's exposure to human-made electromagnetic fields—would have serious consequences. In humans, this would result in tiredness during the day, poor sleep at night, and reduced production of melatonin. All of these effects have been reported in people exposed to continuous, weak, electromagnetic radiation from DECT phone base stations, Wi-Fi routers and cellular antennas.

Also, any weakening of the circadian rhythms' amplitudes means that processes controlled by them will never function at maximum power. The immune system may never be able to summon the massive power that is sometimes required to overcome pathogens or destroy developing cancer cells before they get out of control. In part, this could explain epidemiologists' findings that people living near cellular antennas have an increased cancer risk. It could also explain bee colonies' continuing decreased health and ability to resist pathogens.

Bill Bruno, PhD, biophysicist, retired from the Los Alamos National Lab: *Biology is very sophisticated in its ability to make use of electromagnetic fields. Cryptochromes are just one example. Despite centuries of discoveries in biology and advances in medicine, there is so much we don't know. For example, why do our brains, sinuses and other tissues have magnetic magnetite particles?*

Our bones and collagen are piezoelectric: in an electric field, they expand and contract. What are the implications of that? And what about recent experiments that show that DNA is a semiconductor, and that melanin, including neuromelanin in the brain, is a conductor?

4

Electricity, Magnetics, Electronics, Biology, and the Law: A Summary

Except for light and infrared heat, we can't perceive any of these (radio frequency and other) energies without instruments, so most people don't realize how drastically and abruptly we've changed the electromagnetic environment in just one century.

Robert Becker, MD, *The Body Electric*, 1985

After learning about the brain tumor cluster at SDSU and Veronica Ciandre's experience when cellular antennas were placed on her roof, most people wonder, *How did this happen?* I gave this question to physicists, biologists, and lawyers.

☙

Dr. Gary Olhoeft, a geophysicist and an electrical engineer, worked on the Apollo program and is now professor emeritus at the Colorado School of Mines: His reply considered millions of years of natural evolution, the discovery of electricity, magnetics, electromagnetics, and the electronics revolution: *Our planet is bathed in natural sources of electromagnetic energy, including lightning, the Earth's magnetic field and the fields* *of the sun.*[1] *Please see the glossary for definition of unfamiliar terms.*

Lightning is a visible form of electricity, created when a charge carried by raindrops, winds or dust between clouds and earth produces a voltage difference. When enough difference accumulates, the air breaks down, and the shock of energy (as a huge electrical current) leaps across the gap between clouds and earth. Wind moves charge to create the dry lightning that sometimes causes forest fires. Dust moves charge to create the lightning inside volcanic eruptions, dust storms and explosions in very dry grain storage elevators or coal mines. While walking through dry desert or on a carpet in winter, air accumulates charge, causing a small discharge of electricity when you touch another person or a metal object.

The Earth's magnetic field gives plants, animals and people a compass heading toward north, and also protects us from the particle radiation in the solar wind. Over millions of years, our ecosystem has grown accustomed to this environment. All plants and animals—including humans—have adapted to the Earth's electromagnetic fields, which include a direct current (DC) magnetic field, a DC electrical field and low frequency Schumann Resonances (natural fields that are both electric and magnetic, caused by the geometry of the Earth's surface and the ionosphere near the top of the atmosphere).

When did people begin learning how to store and manipulate electrical energy, then electromagnetic energy—and create electronic technologies? The ancient Greeks knew how to generate electricity, but not store it. In the mid-1600s, the Leyden jar (the first capacitor) was invented to store electricity.

1 National Academy of Sciences, "The Earth's Electrical Environment," Washington, DC: National Academy Press, 1986 p. 263; C. Constable, "Geomagnetic temporal spectrum," *Encyclopedia of Geomagnetism and Paleomagnetism*, D. Gubbins and E. Herrero-Bervera, eds., The Netherlands: Springer, 2005, 353–355.

Around 1800, electricity's biological effects were discovered in the twitching of a frog's legs, which lead to electrochemical battery storage. Once electricity could be generated and stored, manipulation of it through technological applications and electronics followed rapidly.[2]

Around 1750, Ben Franklin discovered that installing a sharply-pointed metal rod with a large cable from the ground through the roof of a house protects the house from harm during a lightning storm: the rod provides a conduit that directs the bolt of electricity into the ground.[3]

Then, starting with the invention of the electromagnet, in 1825, the nineteenth century brought the telegraph (1844), followed by the telephone (1875), and the first power plant (1882). In 1890, Edison's studies of the dangers of electrocution from alternating current (AC) electricity lead to the electric chair, which could put condemned criminals to death.

Inventions such as radio (1890s), the electric washing machine (available in 1904) and the refrigerator (1913) rapidly changed domestic life, created entertainment industries and allowed speedy international communication. The first radio signals crossed the Atlantic in 1901. Military radar first appeared in the 1930s, and, in 1947, the microwave oven, then called "the radar range."

Invention also outpaced regulation.

Since 1897, the National Electric Code (NEC) has codified the requirements for safe electrical installation into a single, standardized source. It is part of the National Fire

---

2 J. F. Keithley, *The Story of Electrical and Magnetic Measurements from 500 BC to the 1940s*, Bangalore, India: IEEE Press, 1999, 240.

3 "Lightning Protection for Engineers," National Lightning Safety Institute, 2009, p. 253; *SOARES Book on Grounding and Bonding*, 10th ed., IAEL, 2008, 429; G. Vijayaraghaven et al, *Practical Grounding, Bonding, Shielding and Surge Protection*, UK: Newnes/Elsevier, 2004, 237.

Code's series published by the National Fire Protection Association (NFPA); and while not itself a U.S. law, NEC use is commonly mandated by state or local zoning laws.[4]

The FCC began regulating the radio spectrum in 1934, mostly to prevent interference in communication.

Sometimes, the benefits of electronic devices brought unintended consequences. For example, emissions from microwave ovens (invented in 1947) frequently interfered with cardiac pacemakers (invented in 1949) and caused the pacemakers to malfunction. But recognition of the problem and consequent Food and Drug Administration (FDA) regulation of microwave ovens did not occur until 1971.[5]

Today, we surround ourselves with radiation-emitting devices, including cordless DECT landline phones, mobile phones, cellular antennas, Wi-Fi, baby monitors, RFID chips and "smart" transmitting utility meters, many of which each operate near the frequency of microwave ovens; and lower frequency power systems, security systems, inventory control systems and many more. Like alternating current (AC) power line electricity, nearly all of these devices operate at frequencies and amplitudes that are often unregulated by any state or federal agency.[6] *Many of these frequencies and amplitudes are not found in nature.*

This leads to the question of the biological effects of human-made electromagnetic energy. In other words, how are plants, animals and humans affected by human-made electricity and wireless devices?

---

4 See www.nema.org/Technical/FieldReps/Documents/NEC-Adoption-Map-PDF.pdf; and NEPA 70 (National Fire Protection Association) 2011, National Electric Code.

5 M. Gruber, ed., *The ARRL RFI Book,* 3rd ed., 2010, var. pp.; see also www.fcc.gov and www.fda.gov.

6 M. Loftness, *AC Power Interference Handbook*, 3rd ed., ARRL, 2007; see http://emfandhealth.com/Science%20Sources.html.

Biological Effects of Human-Made Electricity and Wireless Devices

Before we examine responses to Dr. Olhoeft's question, let me spell out what biologists consider obvious: digesting food, feeling thirsty, locating home, communicating with others, resisting disease, healing infections and broken bones, making decisions, and more are biological functions that depend ultimately on multiple electrical forces.

For a long time, many scientists have believed that human-made electromagnetic fields at routinely encountered frequencies do not disturb biological functioning. Primarily, these scientists have considered the *thermal effects* of exposure to radio frequency (RF) radiation. They recognize that water absorbs radiation, and that the human body is about two thirds water. When the FCC wanted to determine whether cell phones are safe, they gave a two hundred pound anthropomorphic male (a mannequin filled with fluid) a cell phone for six minutes. Because this model head's temperature did not change significantly as a result (the test showed no *thermal* effects), the FCC determined that cell phones are safe.[7]

For decades, however, other researchers have wondered about the *non*-thermal effects of exposure to radio-frequency fields. In 1975, neuroscientist Allan Frey discovered that very weak microwave radiation emitted by Air Force radar (similar to radiation emitted by a cell phone) opens the blood–brain barrier, which provides critical protection for the brain.[8] Dr. Frey also found that microwaves could alter a frog's heart rhythm.

---

7 D. Davis, *Disconnect: The Truth About Cell Phone Radiation, What the Industry is Doing to Hide It, and How to Protect Your Family*, New York: Dutton, 2010.

8 A. H. Frey et al, "Neural function and behavior: Defining the relationship," *Annals of New York Academy of Science,* v. 247 (1975): 433.

Synchronized with the heartbeat, microwave pulses could even stop a frog's heart.[9]

Three and a half decades after Frey published his findings, the *BioInitiative 2012 Report* presents more than 1800 scientific studies that explore the effects of exposure to power lines, common electrical wiring errors, appliances, cordless landlines, mobile phones, cellular antennas, transmitting utility meters, Wi-Fi, baby monitors, and other electronics on DNA, memory, learning, behavior, attention, sleep, cancer, Alzheimer's, and other neurological diseases. (*The BioInitiative Report* also presents solutions.)

According to David O. Carpenter, MD, Professor of Environmental Medicine at SUNY/Albany and coeditor of The *BioInitiative 2012 Report*, "There is now much more evidence of risks to health affecting billions of people worldwide. The status quo is not acceptable in light of the evidence for harm." The *BioInitiative 2012 Report* includes a dozen new studies that link radiation from cell phones to sperm damage. Even a cell phone carried in a pocket or on a belt may harm sperm DNA[10] and impair male fertility. Laptop computers with wireless Internet connections can also damage sperm DNA. Other studies in the *2012 Report* demonstrate that exposure to RF signals from wireless devices increases risk of cancer, neurological diseases, allergies, autism, and more.[11]

RF signals can also interfere with the functioning of medical implants such as cardiac pacemakers, insulin pumps and deep brain stimulators; and these implants have been found to interfere with each other within a person.

In 2011, an agency of the United Nations' World Health Organization (WHO), the International Agency for Research

9 Ibid.

10 C. Sage and D. Carpenter, MD, *BioInitiative Report 2012 press release*, 1-7-2013.

11 Ibid.

on Cancer (IARC), classified radio-frequency fields as "possibly carcinogenic to humans."

As for brain tumors, Swedish oncologist and researcher Lennart Hardell, MD, describes "a consistent pattern of increased risk for glioma [the kind of brain cancer that Rich Farver had] and acoustic neuroma with use of mobile and cordless phones."[12] In the *BioInitiative 2012 Report*, Dr. Hardell explains, "The evidence for risks from prolonged cell phone and cordless phone use is quite strong. For people who have used these devices for ten years or longer, and when they are used mainly on one side of the head, the risk of malignant brain tumor is doubled for adults and is even higher for persons with first use before the age of twenty."

In a letter supporting the Cell Phone Right to Know Act (published in this book's appendix), Thomas K. McInerny, MD, FAAP, President of the American Academy of Pediatrics, wrote, "Children are disproportionately affected by environmental exposures, including cell phone radiation. The differences in bone density and the amount of fluid in a child's brain compared to an adult's brain could allow children to absorb greater quantities of RF (radio frequency) energy deeper into their brains than adults."[13]

Human-made frequency fields also affect wildlife. Dr. Andrew Goldsworthy, professor emeritus of biology at Imperial College in London, says, "Increasing evidence shows that electromagnetic signals from cellular antennas, mobile phones, DECT cordless phones and Wi-Fi interfere with birds' and bees' navigational systems and their circadian (daily) rhythms, which in turn reduces their resistance to disease."

---

12 Ibid.

13 From 12-12-2012 letter to Representative Dennis Kucinich in support of the Cell Phone Right to Know Act.

❦

William Bruno, PhD biophysicist, retired from the Los Alamos National Lab: *Studies show that if someone uses a cell phone before going to sleep, their EEG (brain waves pattern) is slightly altered.*[14] *The nature of change is different in different people, but consistent with the same person. This change in EEG after using a cell phone is significant, because it shows that the brain responds to the cell phone's radiation.*

In 2000, another study showed that steady AC magnetic fields do not disrupt sleep.[15] *But intermittent AC fields—possibly including those created by dirty power and "smart" transmitting utility meters—do disrupt sleep.*

Lots of animal studies show that production of melatonin, a sleep hormone and an important anti-oxidant, is decreased by changes in magnetic field exposure. A slowly varying change does not affect production. But a rapidly varying change (the kind created by magnetic fields) reduces melatonin production.[16]

The quality of one's sleep correlates with overall health. Surrounding ourselves with pulsed electromagnetic fields, including frequencies that disrupt sleep, is not a good idea.

Lots of things are still being discovered. We've just recently learned that near their snouts, dolphins have pores that can

---

14 M.R. Schmid et al, (2012), "Sleep EEG alterations: Effects of different pulse-modulated radio frequency electromagnetic fields," *Journal of Sleep Research*, 21:50–58, doi: 10.1111/j.1365–869. 2011.00918x.

15 C. Graham and M. R. Cook (1999), "Human sleep in 60 Hz magnetic fields," *Bioelectromagnetics*, 20: 277–283, doi: 10:1002/(SICI)1521–186X (1999) 20:5<277:AID-BEM3>3.0.CO:2-U.

16 A. Lerchi et al, (1991), "Pineal gland 'magnetosensitivity' to static magnetic fields is a consequence of induced electric currents (eddy currents)," *Journal of Pineal Research*, 10: 109–116. doi: 10.1111/j.1600–079X.1991.tb00826l.x.

sense weak electric fields[17]*; we already know that sharks, rays, the platypus and the echidna all have an electric sense. Our evolutionary ancestors had such a sense. We know that many animals (and, probably, humans, too) can navigate by using the Earth's magnetic field. In some cases, animals take cues from weaker magnetic deposits underground or undersea. We know that weak fields can have biological effects. Finding all of these effects will take many very careful studies.*

Meanwhile, it's not a stretch to conclude that weak, human-made electromagnetic fields affect melatonin production and sleep, and might easily cause disease over time.

In plain English, over millions of years, we have evolved in relation to electromagnetic energy emitted by the Earth, lightning, and other natural sources. Our cells function by electrochemical signals. Meanwhile, our electrical grid, our appliances, wireless devices and telecommunications equipment function at frequencies and amplitudes (strengths) that are not found in nature. While electricity, appliances, and wireless devices keep us efficient and entertained, they emit electromagnetic radiation; and these emissions have the ability to affect basic biological functioning, including our ability to sleep.

Call these inconvenient truths. We could close the conversation here. Or, we could explore these issues in more depth—and find solutions.

Consider this book an invitation to anyone whose life is affected by electricity, appliances, and wireless communications to name their questions and observations and join this discussion.

---

17 D. Czech-Damal et al, "Electroreception in the Guiana dolphin (*Sotalia guianensis*)," *Proceedings of the Royal Society,* B2012 279, doi;10.1098/rspb.2011.1127.

The Law

Before learning how electricity gets to your house, what magnetic fields and broadband over power lines are, how using a cell phone can lead to brain cancer (etc.), we've got another issue to put on the table: the legal situation. As it is, our rules and regulations value telecommunications above our health and environment. Our human-made laws do not consider nature's laws.

Here's an example: The Telecommunications Act (the TCA), which Congress passed in 1996, actually *prohibits* municipalities from protecting their community's health or ecosystem. The TCA's Section 704 states, "No state or local government or instrumentality thereof may regulate the placement, construction, or modification of personal wireless service facilities on the basis of the environmental effects of radio frequency emissions." In this case, "environmental effects" includes health effects.

In other words, according to federal law, no health or environmental concern may interfere with the placement of telecommunications equipment.

Here's another example: if a manufacturer wants to sell a new electronic device, they must prove to the Federal Communications Commission (FCC) that the product (perhaps a mobile phone, a security device, a baby monitor, a Wi-Fi router) does not interfere with existing radio, TV, or Internet broadcasts. To comply with the FCC's safety regulations, the manufacturer only has to prove that the device does not heat body tissue significantly after a few minutes of exposure. These are the "thermal effects" described earlier. Even though thousands of studies have identified *non*-thermal effects from exposure to radiation emitted by wireless devices, the FCC does not recognize them. In the U.S., no agency does.

Let's return to this question: *How did San Diego State's cancer cluster happen?* After President Clinton signed the Telecom

Act of 1996 into law, the telecommunications industry initiated a massive advertising campaign. With corporations free to develop and market services and devices regardless their impact on our health or ecosystem, and with no agency authorized to study the biological effects of such services or devices or to warn us about the risks of using them, almost all of us tried mobile devices and Wi-Fi—and got hooked. Thrilled by all that technology enables us to do, we subscribed en masse to it, excluding health or environmental concerns from our awareness.

Since wireless devices can't operate without a base station, most of us now live, work, and attend school (like Rich Farver did) near cellular antennas—as well as transmitting utility meters. As we increase our demand for online video (which requires more data and thus more broadband), we increase demand for more antennas—and expose ourselves to more electromagnetic radiation.

As the questions continue, let's clarify what we can and cannot control. We (society, government agencies, industry, businesses, individuals) cannot change the Earth's electromagnetic energy. Electronic devices add to our environmental spectrum of electromagnetic energy. Building a shielded room may reduce exposure to RF radiation and lower frequency fields; but this may also block exposure to the Earth's electromagnetic fields. We cannot change our biological responses to electromagnetic fields. *Do we have the will to change our rules and regulations and reduce our exposure to radiation? Do we have the will to change our thinking and behavior?*

5

What's New Under Heaven?

Without Dr. Gary Olhoeft, geophysicist, electrical engineer and patient teacher, this chapter would not be.

He unleashes His lightning beneath the whole heaven
and sends it to the ends of the earth.
After that... God's voice thunders in marvelous ways;
He does great things beyond our understanding.
Job 37:3–5

Part One: Human-made Electricity

Before we learn how mobile phones and other wire*less* devices work, we need to know how electricity gets delivered through wires.

Let me repeat that simplifying descriptions of electricity—which I do throughout this book—can make the information slightly inaccurate. I am not writing a manual for engineers or electricians. I aim to give laypersons (like myself) a vocabulary for further education and discussion. For more comprehensive descriptions of electricity, please check out physics textbooks written for high school or first-year college students.

Electrical Fundamentals

All matter is made from about one hundred and eighteen elements. The smallest particle of an element is an *atom*. An atom is made up of *electrons*, which carry a negative charge, *protons*, which carry a positive charge, and *neutrons*, which are electrically neutral. (For this discussion, protons and neutrons are not important, although they would be for MRIs, radioactive decay, and more.)

An electron's or proton's charge creates an electrical field. Electrical fields cause forces that make charged particles move. Like charges repel. Their fields create forces that make them move away from each other. Unlike charges (one negative and one positive) attract. Their forces move them toward each other. Electrically charged objects exert a force on each other. This force causes them to move.

Moving electrons are called an *electrical current*. Charge separation and discharge (discussed later) both require moving electrons. An electron in motion also creates a magnetic field. A magnetic field that changes with time exerts a force on charged particles just like an electrical field, also causing them to move.

An electron changing speed radiates an electromagnetic field that changes with time. Electrons interacting between atoms create chemical bonds and thus molecules, most chemistry, and chemical reactions.

Lightning is an electrical charge separation. It happens when charge builds up between clouds and the Earth's surface. Wind or rainfall carry charges to the surface, separating them as negative charges in the clouds attract to the positively charged ground. When sufficient charge accumulates, the atmosphere breaks down, and a large current flow discharges, restoring the original cloud-ground charge equilibrium. This discharge of current flow heats the air (to as much as 20,000 degrees Centigrade) and creates a streak of light and loud sound that we call lightning and thunder.[1] A lightning bolt is a cloud-to-ground discharge, a huge current that also creates a huge magnetic field.

---

1 T. Hsu, *Integrated Science: An Investigative Approach,* Peabody, MA: CPO Science, 2007.

Similarly, other forces can separate charges, accumulate them or charge an object. Your body can accumulate charges—then discharge them. For example, if you rub your feet on carpet on a dry day, then touch something metallic like a doorknob, you'll feel an electrical shock, which is an electrical discharge. Brushing your hair on a dry day can also generate electrical charge separation.

Electricity

Electricity includes natural phenomena (like lightning) and human-made technologies (like the 60 Hz available at wall outlets). Electricity can be delivered two ways:

Direct current (DC) electricity flows only in one direction, from positive to negative terminals. It occurs with constant polarity and constant amplitude with no time variation. Direct current creates a constant amplitude current and a static or DC magnetic field. It does not oscillate. A battery is a good example of a DC source of electricity.

With *alternating current (AC)* electricity, the current flows between positive and negative polarities that oscillate in time: the electrons move back and forth in the wire, creating a wave in space and time. The oscillation is a frequency, measured in hertz.

Hertz (Hz) is the number of complete cycles that occurs per second. Hertz is a measure of frequency.

AC occurs with an amplitude (strength) that varies in time from zero to a maximum positive amplitude peak, back through zero to a maximum negative peak, and back to zero—which constitutes one cycle, which then repeats. This cycle looks like a wave, where a rope swung by two people looks like half of a wave.

Usually, over long distances, alternating current transmits electricity with less loss (with more energy efficiency) than direct current. AC also allows transformers within the grid to change voltage easily. AC also allows wireless induced current charging of some battery operated devices (such as electric toothbrushes, electric shavers, cell phones and cameras).

Electrical Circuits

A circuit is a circle. An open circuit cannot deliver an electrical impulse because it has a break in the circle. A closed circuit can deliver electricity, because it has no breaks. If you turn a light switch *off*, you've got an *open* circuit: electricity cannot access the lightbulb. If you turn the switch *on*, then you've got an electrical circuit, a closed loop. Electricity will flow to your lightbulb and light your room, then flow back to its source, closing the loop.

Your nervous system is also a network of electrical circuits that includes your brain, spinal cord and many nerves. In order to move, your motor nerves send electrical messages to your muscles that tell them to contract. If a motor nerve gets injured, say in your pointer finger, then your finger won't receive your brain's messages, and your finger's muscles won't work: the electrical circuit from your brain to your finger will be blocked.[2]

Characteristics of Electricity

Let's go over the terms that describe electricity:

Frequency refers to the cyclical change of voltage or current and the number of waves or oscillations that occur in one second in AC electricity. These cycles per second are called *hertz* (Hz). Electricity is typically delivered in North America at 60 Hz, in Europe at 50 Hz, and in airplanes at 400 Hz. If hertz reaches the kilohertz (kHz) range—thousands of cycles per second—it creates radio frequency (RF) electromagnetic radiation. Microwaves begin at 300 megahertz (MHz), 300 million cycles per second. Wireless devices use microwaves; we'll discuss them in part two of this chapter.

---

2 Ibid.

Voltage measures the amplitude (strength) of electrical pressure (or potential) that makes charge move. The electrical potential in volts causes electrons to move and create a current when a switch is turned on. Electrical potential is like water pressure in a pipe: no water flows until a valve opens to release pressure. Electrical current will not flow until a switch is turned on. In the U.S., most household outlets operate at 120 volts AC. Ovens and dryers usually operate at 240 volts AC. European outlets typically operate at 230 volts AC. Most cars, trucks, boats and RVs operate at 12 or 24 volts DC.

Amperes (or Amps) refers to the strength of an electrical current. Amperes measure the flow in a cable, similar to water in a pipe.

A watt is a unit of power. Volts times amperes equals power in watts, and consumption of electricity is measured in watt-hours or watts times hours of use.

Fields are characterized by their amplitude variations in space and time. Electric fields are measured in Volts per meter; magnetic fields are measured in amperes per meter.

Wavelength A wavelength is defined by the speed of light and the frequency. It is measured in meters, in space. The lower a frequency, the longer a wavelength. Wavelength = speed of light in meters per second divided by frequency in cycles per second. A wavelength is a meter per cycle.

Phase AC electricity is sometimes phased, which shifts it in time in order to keep the return wire running the same amount of current all the time.

Getting Electricity to Your House

Typically, AC electricity arrives at your house (and returns to its source at the power generating station) by three cabled loops. The first loop starts at the (coal, nuclear, hydro, solar or wind) power generating station and goes to the substation transformer—and returns to the power generating station. The second loop circles from the substation to your neighborhood transformer—and back. The third loops circles from your neighborhood's transformer to your house—and back.

Let's return to the power generating station, which regulates the electrical current's frequency and voltage, then sends it to a substation through an assemblage of high tension wires, circuit breakers, disconnect switches and transformers. Transmission lines (also called high tension lines) typically carry high voltages of 230,000 volts or more to bring current from the power plant to the substation and back to the power plant.

At the substation, *transformers* lower the 230,000 volts to 1,000 volts, and distribute electricity on power lines to small transformers that are mounted on utility poles throughout a neighborhood. (A transformer reduces or increases voltage using magnetic coils of wire.) These transformers on utility poles look like small, metal trash cans, and they typically have circuit breakers.

Besides holding transformers, utility poles also hold up primary distribution lines. (As rentable space, they may also hold phone or cable TV wires or internet fiber optics.) These wires may also be buried underground. A neighborhood transformer, which serves about five households, reduces voltage to the 120/240 volts needed in each home.

Electricity arrives at a house's meter, which is usually located outside of the house and connected to the circuit breaker panel. There are two kinds of meters: one is analog mechanical. The other is digital electronic. Placing a digital, wireless, transmitting meter (a "smart" meter) on homes, schools and businesses may generate high frequencies on wires that harm health and wildlife. (This issue is discussed in other chapters.) The circuit breaker panel's placement depends on local zoning code. Code is usually governed by the National Electric Code (NEC), which is voluntary. "Smart" meter transmissions may also be regulated by the FCC.

To complete the three loops, power will return from a building's circuit breaker panel through a neutral wire to the transformer on the neighborhood utility pole, then to the substation, and finally to the power generating plant.

Wiring in a Circuit Panel Box

The circuit panel box has several kinds of wires:

- two "hot" wires that are insulated in red or black cable; on these wires, the current enters your house from your neighborhood's transformer.
- a "neutral" wire, also called the "return" wire, usually in a white, insulated cable; it *returns* current to your neighborhood transformer.
- a "ground" wire—it'll be bare or covered with green insulation; it attaches to a ground bus. The ground bus is bonded to the back of the panel box and to the neutral bus (which connects to the power company's neutral). If an appliance short circuits, enough current will (hopefully) flow from that circuit's hot wire through the ground bus, then back to the power company's neutral to trip that breaker in your panel, prevent an electrical fire and protect people in the house from getting shocked.
- a "ground" rod, usually a six-foot metal rod (or, copper plumbing pipes, or both) connects the electrical system to earth. In dry environments, it's very difficult to get a good ground-to-earth connection. In wet environments, rapid metallic corrosion may negate the ground over time. If the ground is not functioning properly, ground currents (or in a marina, currents in water) may cause a fire, shock or electrocution hazard.

A ground wire also runs from your breaker box to each outlet. If your wiring is correct, it carries negligible current. In case the neutral does not work, the ground provides an alternate return path. Most outlets near water (in bathrooms, kitchens, garages marinas and outdoors) have ground-fault circuit interrupters (GFCIs), which switch off quickly if they detect current going to ground instead of through the neutral wire. Since 1999, new houses are also required to have an Arc Fault Circuit Interrupter (AFCI) in bedrooms. It prevents sparks that cause fires.

Electric and Magnetic Fields

Wherever there is electricity, there are electric fields and magnetic fields. They emit radiation (discussed in later sections). Normally, electric and magnetic fields occur together and are called electromagnetic fields (EMFs). EMFs generated by power lines might extend for many miles, while those generated by a refrigerator might extend a few feet. Usually, EMFs are invisible and inaudible.

Electrical current in power lines, lights and appliances produces electric fields. Strong electric fields sometimes produce a crackling noise or buzzing—or a shock.

Electrical current also generates magnetic fields. The higher the current, the stronger the magnetic field. Magnetic fields are measured in units called gauss (G), tesla (T) or amperes per meter (A/m). Because one of these units is *extremely* large, engineers usually measure magnetic fields in milligauss (mG) or microtesla (uT).

Properly installed, hot wires (that deliver electricity) and neutral wires (that return the current to its source) are twisted together to cancel the magnetic field that results from the current flow in each loop.

What else creates magnetic fields? Transformers, electric motors, induction charging systems, "smart" appliances, and digital electronics (including mobile phones, cameras, tablets, laptops, TVs, and electric wheelchairs) can generate magnetic fields. If the current returns to the ground, the magnetic fields are not canceled. The neutral wire must return to the breaker box, and current should not flow through the ground wire or through plumbing.[3]

Errors on the utility company's equipment can also cause problems: a loose bolt on supporting hardware for a power distribution transmission line can generate tiny sparks. Any spark contains a wide range of frequencies; including some that go up to the hundreds of megahertz. Ham radio operators know this radio noise very well. These sparks can cause radio interference up to a half mile away. Power line sparking also depends on the air's moisture content and temperature. Dry air will allow sparks to happen more easily; but after rain, wet, wooden utility poles can actually tighten the loose connections temporarily.

Magnetic or electric fields can create health and safety problems. Long-term exposure to even low levels of magnetic fields increases the risk of childhood leukemia[4] and other diseases (see chapter 4).

You need a magnometer to identify magnetic fields. A portable, AM radio can work as a crude meter (see the appendices).

Stray/Ground Current

If a utility company sends 10 kilowatts (k/W) of electricity to a home or building, those 10 k/Ws will return to their power source—or you won't have an electric current. Again, this is like the flow of water: water comes in by pipes and goes out by

3 K. Riley, *Tracing EMFs in Building Wiring and Grounding, 2nd ed.,* Acton, MA: Magnetic Sciences, 2005.

4 S. Greenland et al, "A pooled analysis of magnetic fields, wire codes, and childhood leukemia," *Epidemiology,* 11 (2000): 624–634.

the sewer system. Shutting a valve or turning a switch off stops the flow.

"Stray" currents form when the return current is allowed a second or multiple pathway(s) (such as on metal plumbing pipes) back to the transformer. Stray current is like a leak in a water pipe.

Ground current can occur anywhere that electricity is delivered. It was first identified in the 1940s, when electricity was installed in rural areas. Ground current can be deadly. If someone showers in a stall whose pipe is not properly grounded, steps off of a boat that is not properly grounded or swims in a pool with stray currents, they can be electrocuted.

According to "Worker Deaths by Electrocution," a 1998 report by the National Institute for Occupational Safety and Health (NIOSH), more than four hundred people die annually by electrocution on the job, making electrocution the fifth leading cause of death on the job.

What makes a good ground bad? Wet, muddy (acidic) dirt—like that found in moist climates—can corrode a metal grounding rod quickly. In dry climates, it's harder to locate a good ground; but once found, it lasts longer. If you have a bad ground, chances of getting ground current and/or dirty power increase.

Our (voluntary) national electrical codes may actually prevent safe delivery of electricity. In a paper given at the Institute of Electrical and Electronics Engineers (IEEE) in 1999, "Are the National Electrical Code and the National Electrical Safety Code Hazardous to Your Health?," electrical engineer Donald W. Zipse described a shocking swimming pool in a condominium complex. He explained that swimmers can be shocked because of NESC codes that save utilities money but create hazardous conditions. For example, the NESC requires utilities to connect the primary neutral to the secondary neutral in distribution transformers; permits the neutral and ground conductors to be combined in one conductor; and requires multiple connections to earth. Further, utilities often install neutral cables without any protective jacket. These practices encourage "the flow of continuous, uncontrolled current over the earth, metal piping, building steel, etc." and can result in electrical shocks to humans and livestock. European countries prohibit such practices.

ꕥ

Don Hillman, PhD, Professor Emeritus of Animal Science, Michigan State University: *Numerous times, I've observed cows refuse to enter their barns at milking time because of electrical ground currents. Cows have four feet and no rubber soles. If, for example, the milking machine is not properly grounded, when a cow picks up one foot, her resistance changes, and she gets a greater shock. If she remains exposed to ground currents, she becomes part of the circuit and will get shocked frequently.*

Ground current also reduces milk production. I've seen many cows die and many farmers go out of business because of it.

In 2003, Dr. Hillman presented papers about dairy cattle and electricity to the American Society of Agricultural Engineers, the American Dairy Science Association, and the Canadian Agricultural and Food Science Engineers. They're available at electricalpollution.com.

Dirty Power, Damaged Electronics, Wasted Energy and Health

When electrical equipment malfunctions because of ground problems, high amplitude spikes and/or transients on wires, engineers call the source of the problem "excessive harmonics," "high frequency content" or "dirty power." Meanwhile, some devices, such as fluorescent bulbs, dimmer switches and some battery chargers create dirty power when they function "properly."

Dirty power proves costly: besides damaging equipment, it wastes energy. BC Hydro, a western Canadian electric company, *charges* its business customers a surcharge if their equipment causes too much dirty power.[5]

Dirty power can also affect human health. Ed Leeper, a physicist, and Nancy Wertheimer, a Colorado epidemiologist, were among the first people to identify health problems caused by dirty power's magnetic fields. In the 1970s, Dr. Wertheimer wondered why 344 children in her state had died of cancer. After driving around Denver, she noticed that many of the homes of children who had died were near pole-mounted electrical transformers. In the last two years of their lives, a significant percentage of the young leukemia victims in Colorado had been exposed to magnetic fields.[6]

Epidemiologist Dr. Samuel Milham's book, *Dirty Electricity*, reports several other cancer clusters caused by dirty power.

Some Events that Generate High-Frequency Fields, Harmonics, Arcing, and Transient Noise—which Emit Electromagnetic Radiation (EMR)

Note: we are discussing non-ionizing, non-particle electromagnetic radiation below 300 GHz.

Natural events:

Lightning

Ground currents generated by the sun's solar wind impacting the Earth's magnetic field.

---

5 See www.bchydro.com/powersmart/technology_tips/harmonics.html; www.bchydro.com/etc/medialib/internet/documents/psbusiness/pdf/; and Power_Factor.Par.001.File.Power_Factor.pdf.

6 N. Wertheimer and Ed Leeper, "Electrical wiring configurations and childhood cancer," *American Journal of Epidemiology*, 109 (1979): 273–284; also E. Sugarman, *Warning: The Electricity Around You May Be Hazardous to Your Health*, Whitby, ON: Fireside, 1992.

Tree branches contacting high voltage wires.

Repairable faults in the system:

Loose connections, especially on the high voltage side of the transformer.

Wiring errors such as paired neutrals.

Properly designed electronics that transmit/radiate unintentionally:

Switch-mode power supplies.

Fluorescent lights, including compact fluorescents (CFLs).

Dimmer switches and touch-lamps.

Induction chargers for battery powered devices (mobile phones, laptops, tablets, cameras, electric toothbrushes, shavers, arc welders, etc.).

High-voltage power lines.

Digital equipment:

Digital, transmitting, wireless "smart" utility meters.

Digital electronics and appliances, including "smart" and energy-saving appliances.

Digital modulated TV and radio, and all mobile phones.

Types of Electromagnetic Radiation

The preceding list presents some *sources* of EMR. Here are some *types* of EMR. Again, we're discussing non-ionizing, non-particle electromagnetic radiation below 300 GHz:

Induced EMR: a time-varying magnetic field or a low-frequency magnetic field induces a current in a conductor, inside a wire. A transformer is a common example.

Conducted EMR: where an electromagnetic wave rides on the outside of a conductor. Examples are TVs and laptops that have a bump on the cord near the device; this "ferrite" absorbs conducted energy and prevents it from following the wire.

Radiated EMR: radio and TV broadcasts, which occur through the air.

Sound radiation occurs for any particle movement. EMR only occurs for charged particle movement.

Anything digital or pulsed generates all three kinds of EMR and may also generate sound radiation.

Transformers and Power Supplies

Electronics (i.e., computers, printers, battery chargers, devices with a digital display) operate on direct current (DC) electricity at low voltages. To access the alternating current (AC) electricity available at standard wall outlets, electronics also require a transformer, which is part of the device's "power supply." Like neighborhood transformers that reduce voltage so that electricity can be delivered safely to your home, an electronic device's power supply reduces the voltage with a voltage regulator and a capacitor. Its rectifier makes the current go only in one direction and converts the AC to DC electricity. Its filter smooths the current.

Even when a device is turned off (but plugged into an outlet), the power supply pulls electrical current in short bursts and "chops it up," creating electronic "hash" or "noise" on your wiring.

Further, TVs, electronic alarm clocks, energy efficient washing machines, and energy efficient heating and cooling systems (with variable speed motors)—and computers, printers, fluorescent lights, cell phone chargers, and countless other electronics—use electricity in *pulses*, rather than in a smooth, continuous current. Pulsed signals chop current, radiating EMFs, and increasing opportunities for biological effects.

Before 2000, electronics commonly had linear power supplies. These looked like black bricks on the devices' electric cords. Since 2000, we've had switch-mode power supplies

(SMPSs), usually installed *within* a device. Compared to linear power supplies, SMPSs waste less energy as heat. In addition to chopping up current, an SMPS's transformer also generates a high-frequency square wave.

⌘

Bill Bruno, PhD, biophysicist: *Switch-mode power supplies generate high frequency square waves that have harmonics going up to many megahertz. These radio frequency pulses end up on electrical wiring. An oscilloscope can best detect these harmonics. You can hear them more affordably with a portable, analog AM radio. Lower frequency harmonics (in the kilohertz frequencies) can be heard with a magnetic pickup (aka a "telephone listener") plugged into a speaker (available on eBay or at lessemfs.com).*

If the SMPS operates above 1.5 MHz, it won't show up on an AM radio, but it can be heard on an Airband radio that tunes in to air traffic.

We don't know the biological implications of exposure to square waves at multiple frequencies. But research from cardiovascular surgeon William Rea, MD[7] *shows that people do react to square waves. They can tell whether or not they're near high frequencies. The sudden changes in field at the beginning and end of a square wave pulse may confuse biological signaling, which is largely based on sudden spikes in voltage.*

Convincing the many skeptics about this issue will require research—and that will require funding.

Lighting

Because fluorescent lights (including CFLs) need higher voltage than the 120 volts available in our homes, schools, and offices, they have a *ballast* that increases the voltage available for the

7 W. J. Rea et al, "Electromagnetic field sensitivity," *Journal of Bioelectricity,* vol. 10 (1991): nos. 1 and 2, 243–256.

bulb. Sometimes, people could see earlier models of fluorescent bulbs (using older ballasts) flicker 120 times per second. Newer fluorescents, using electronic ballasts (which operate similarly to SMPSs), flicker 30,000 times per second. We can't see this flickering, although some people may react to it. For a description of flicker-sensitivity, go to conradbiologic.com.

Fluorescents also use a heating element to vaporize the mercury inside each bulb. The bulbs use high voltage to create ultra violet light. The coating inside of the bulb "fluoresces" and turns the UV into visible white light. If the bulb's coating gets scratched, looking at its ultra violet light can burn and hurt the viewer's eyes. Wikipedia has a more comprehensive description.

Dimmer switches and touch lamps also contribute to dirty power. So can switches that let you turn a light off or on from more than one switch if they are not properly installed.

Use incandescent lights as much as possible. (May their production be restored.) Large stores and gymnasiums concerned about reducing employees' and patrons' exposure to flickering and square waves might use 12 volt DC LEDs (*not* fluorescents or halogens with SMPSs or RF lights).

Wind- and Solar-Powered Electricity

Because of climate changes and other issues, many conscientious people have turned to wind or solar powered electricity as a partial solution to reduce their use of fossil fuels. They may be unaware of the dirty power typically generated by such systems.

Modern wind turbines create variable (*not* 60 Hz) frequency AC signals. Variable frequency sine waves from wind turbines are first rectified to create direct current. An inverter then converts the DC from wind turbines (or solar panels) to standard AC power (60 Hz) that can be distributed on the grid. The conversion process creates dirty power. Charge controllers and other components can also create dirty power.

Some inverters take DC and create a pure 60 Hz sine wave with no harmonics, such as some uninterruptable power supplies for sensitive electronics. (Uninterruptable power supplies are used by some computers, which can be damaged if they're exposed to "noise" and non-pure sine waves and/or abrupt on-off switches.) Inverters that do not create a pure 60 Hz sine wave can create harmonics and/or dirty power.

Windfall, a documentary, presents the experience of people who installed wind turbines on their property and later regretted it.

Other Voices on Electricity and Magnetic Fields

Sonia Hoglander, electrical engineer, MBA, building biology consultant, Washington: *In 2005, I measured my house's magnetic fields with a gauss meter; the levels didn't alarm me. In August, 2012, I took readings again. Every room measured between 1.2 mG and 1.8 mG. I turned off my fuse box, and still, even on the second floor, some rooms measured 1.2 mG.*

Exposure to chronic, low-level magnetic fields causes sleep disturbances. Is my insomnia caused by the magnetic fields in my house?

I asked my utility company to send an engineer to identify the source of my magnetic fields. At my neighborhood transformer, she found that the levels measured lower than they did at my house. The engineer and I scratched our heads. Then, in the driveway of a neighbor who has children, the magnetic fields measured higher than they did at my house. In the trees about 150 feet from my house, the engineer and I saw 230 kV power lines that I'd never noticed before. At about 150 feet, a 230 kV power line is consistent with a magnetic field of 1.2 mG.

I became alarmed. Milligauss readings above 1.0 are especially hazardous for children, pregnant women, people with medical implants and those with compromised health.

The engineer said, "Let me allay your fears. My house reads over 2 mG. All of these levels are far *from the federal limit, which is 1000 mG. If you had children, you might be concerned. But you don't have children."*

Her words did not allay my fears.

In my experience, correcting wiring errors, moving beds and work stations, and shielding key rooms may provide some relief for some people. But these are Band-Aids for an antiquated electrical system. And shielding high frequencies, for example, may intensify the effects of magnetic fields. I'm an electrical engineer and a building biologist, and I cannot remedy the problems at my own house.

We need to learn how to identify the sources of these fields and how to eliminate them. We need to quit wireless devices, return to cabled ones and *reduce our use of electricity. Transitioning will inconvenience every single person. But what is the alternative?*

ஐ

Don Hillman, PhD, Professor Emeritus of Animal Science, Michigan State: *At my house, which was built in 1967, the neutral wire attaches to copper water pipes. Decades ago, when electrical codes were written for the safe installation of electrical systems, authorities obviously did not expect that a household would use electricity in ways we now consider normal. Unfortunately, in 2013 neutral wires bear more current than they were intended to handle. Furthermore, our electrical code has not been updated to meet our changed use of electricity.*

In my house, the neutral wire runs along the basement's ceiling, below our first floor. My gauss meter measured up to 50 mG in the living room. Electricians came and measured near the water pipe and beside the neutral wire in the basement. They measured between 280 and 320 mG—quite alarming, though well within our federal limit of 1000 mG.

Our utility company sent engineers to resolve the problem at my house. Nothing made a difference until they cut our copper water pipe and inserted a dielectric coupling (a small, plastic tube with rubber insulation inside), that broke the current and reduced the mG rate to nearly zero.

Unfortunately, my neighbors did not receive attention. Those with plastic PEX water pipes have less of a problem; but everyone is still affected. Now, our utility company plans to install "smart" meters. I will testify that we are not prepared for more high frequencies on our already severely compromised grid.

⌘

Gary Olhoeft, PhD, geophysicist and electrical engineer: *There's a lot of disagreement about how to address electrical problems, especially since we're all connected now in one big grid.*

To begin, we need to revise our electrical code so that every dwelling, school, office building, hospital and factory gets reviewed at least every five years. Electricians need to see if loose connections, corrosion of connections and ground rods, "smart" meters, broadband over power lines or other problems are reducing power quality. Devices that harm power quality will need to be removed—or filters will need to isolate the noisy device from the clean devices. (Typically, filters are needed at the breaker box between the noisy power line and "smart" meter and the clean house power—but also possibly between each noisy device in the house.)

In Europe, some engineers are replacing the existing electrical system with a healthier one. We North Americans need to pay attention: our survival depends on using electricity safely and by drastically reducing our use of it.

Part Two: Radio-Frequency Fields

In alternating current (AC) electricity, *hertz* (the frequency of cycles per second) causes electrons to accelerate and decelerate. When oscillations reach *kilohertz* (kHz)—thousands of cycles per second—they create radio frequency (RF) electromagnetic radiation. We use RFs to operate radio stations, mobile phones, cellular antennas, "smart" digital transmitting utility meters—and microwave ovens. Microwaves, which begin at 300 MHz (300 million cycles per second), are a kind of radio frequency field.

How Charge Moves

Diffusion occurs at lower frequencies. Flipping a light switch makes charge move by diffusion. Diffusing a field at a lower frequency is like dropping a rock into mud: the first ripple dies. In the diffusion domain, a radio transmitter would transmit for half a meter or less. *Induction* is the electromagnetic term meaning diffusion, and generally occurs at low frequencies, below the kilohertz.

Propagation of the electromagnetic field results from charge accelerating or decelerating. To make charge accelerate or decelerate, you need to store it, which creates the possibility of radiation. Dropping a rock into a pond makes ripples that go away from the rock and creates something that looks like propagation. Propagation usually occurs at higher frequencies, generally above the kilohertz. A cell phone operates by propagation. So does a radio station.

To broadcast a music or talk show, a radio station must *transmit* a frequency. Say it's 101.1 FM. "101.1" stands for 101.1 megahertz (MHz)-101.1 million oscillations per second. When you tune your radio to 101.1 FM, it *receives* that station's frequency. On top of that base carrier frequency is encoded the information content by a modulation: amplitude modulation

(AM radio) frequency modulation (FM radio), pulse code modulation (PCM), and so forth.

The Electromagnetic Frequency Spectrum

The electromagnetic (EM) spectrum organizes EM fields by the frequency of their oscillations. While physicists likely would agree with these definitions, electrochemists might find them inadequate, since they typically consider a field's amplitude as important as its frequency. Biochemists consider a field's duration as important as its frequency.

The *non-ionizing* EM spectrum (categorized only by frequency) starts with zero oscillations and extends to hundreds of trillions of oscillations per second, which is visible light. *Ionizing* radiation starts with frequencies of oscillation above visible light. X-rays and gamma rays are ionizing. When ionizing radiation is emitted or absorbed by an atom, it can liberate a particle (usually an electron) from the atom.

For example, based on frequency alone, lightning is non-ionizing. But because a lightning strike's amplitude is so high, it ionizes the atmosphere and also produces heat and light.

The International Telecommunications Union meets periodically to allocate different portions of the frequency spectrum between countries for radio, TV, and Internet broadcasts, as well as geographical instruments, radio astronomy, first responder radio, and military radio. Within each country, regulatory agencies control use of the spectrum. In the U.S., the FCC and the National Telecommunications and Information Agency (NTIA) control and regulate spectrum use.

The Ionizing and Non-ionizing Frequency Spectrum

This spectrum does not include amplitude, duration, or modulation, which also affect electromagnetic energy.

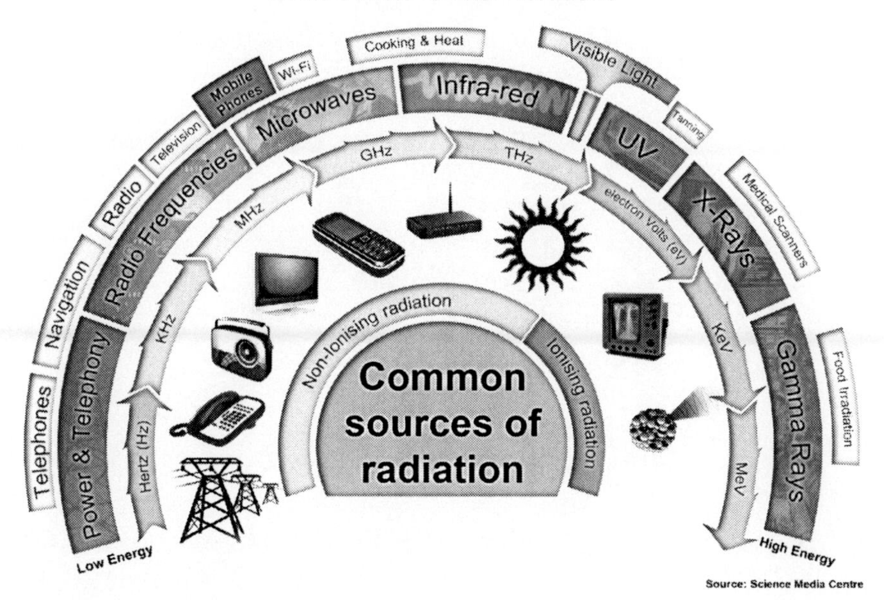

Extra Low Frequencies (ELFs) extend from just above zero to 3 kHz, 3,000 cycles per second. The natural fields of the Earth and Sun, our heart, brain, and other organs operate at ELFs. So does our 60 Hz electrical grid.

Very Low Frequencies extend from 3 kHz to 300,000 cycles per second (300 kHz). Many switch-mode power supplies (for modern appliances and other electronics) operate at these frequencies.

High Frequencies extend from 300 kHz to 300 megahertz, or 300 MHz. Radio and TV broadcasts operate in this range.

Microwave Frequencies extend from 300 MHz (300 million cycles per second) to 300 gigahertz (GHz; 300 billion cycles per second). Wireless devices like cordless landline phones, cell phones and transmitting utility meters, and services like Wi-Fi and broadband over power lines operate in this range.

Terrahertz waves (around one trillion hertz) are used in new airport scanners.

Infra-red (everything between terahertz and visible light, which is found at the hundreds of trillions of hertz) is used for a TV's remote control and military night-vision technology.

The Frequencies of Some Electronic Devices

- The U.S. electrical grid operates at 60 Hz; it also generates harmonics at frequencies that include 120 Hz, 180 Hz, 240 Hz, 300 Hz and so on.
- Metal detectors at airports, libraries, federal buildings, and malls operate at 100 to 3,500 Hz.
- A deep brain stimulator (medical implant for people with Parkinson's) runs between 130 and 185 Hz.
- An airplane's power system runs at 400 Hz.
- TV broadcasts use "very high frequency" (VHF) waves, above 54 MHz. "Ultra-high frequency" (UHF) channels use up to 800 MHz.
- AM (amplitude modulation) radio uses about 500 to 1,600 kHz, also known as 0.5 to1.6 MHz, to transmit music or speech. AM can pick up lightning bolts; FM cannot.
- FM (frequency modulation) radio uses 88 MHz to 108 MHz.
- In the U.S., mobile phones may use one or more of the following frequency bands to operate: 700 MHz, 800 MHz, 850 MHz, 900 MHz, 1,700 MHz, 1,800 MHz, 1,900 MHz, 2,100 MHz and 2,500 MHz. In other countries, mobile phones may use one or more of the following frequency bands: 450 MHz, 480 MHz, 860 MHz, 900 MHz, 1,700 MHz, 1,800 MHz, 1,900 MHz, 2,300 MHz and 2,400 MHz.
- DECT (Digital Enhanced Cordless Telecommunications) phones also use two frequency bands, 1,900 MHz and 1,980 MHz.
- A microwave oven operates at 2.4 GHz (2.4 billion oscillations per second).
- Most wireless Internet connections (Wi-Fi) use 2.4GHz or higher.
- "Smart" meters (digital utility meters) operate at frequencies between 900 to 928 MHz (for the carrier wave) and at 2.4 GHz (for the data wave).
- New body scanners at airports operate at frequencies above 300 GHz.

Devices that operate at a similar frequency may interfere with each other's functioning more strongly than devices with frequencies that are farther apart. Again, amplitude, duration and modulation matter.

Transmitting Voice and Pictures on Phones

To speak and hear on corded landline phones, voices are converted to signals that travel through cables at low frequencies whose radiation emissions do not reach far past the cable or the handset. Wire*less* devices now typically use digital, pulsed modulated signals; they carry data that encodes a person's voice from, say, the mobile phone to a cellular antenna network, and then to the phone that receives the call.

Sending a photo requires more data than sending the voice. Sending the voice requires more data than a text message. A video requires more data than any of these.

The more electromagnetic oscillations that occur in one second (the higher the hertz), the more data can be transmitted.

Mobile devices also require more than one microwave frequency to function, which makes them modulated. For example, AT&T's voice frequencies operate in the 850 and 1,900 MHz bands. The 850 Hz band is uplinked (used for outgoing voice) at 824.2. to 849.0 MHz. The downlink side (used for voice coming toward you) is 869.2 to 894.0 MHz.

Speaking, sending a text, using Wi-Fi, using Bluetooth—and receiving each of these—each requires a different frequency. Doing more than one of these activities at a time requires multiple frequencies. Different providers (i.e., AT&T, Sprint, Verizon) each use different frequencies for their services.[8]

Electromagnetic signals for mobile phones, cordless phones, "smart" meters, baby monitors, Wi-Fi, GPS networks, and

8 For more on how cell phones work, go to www.electronics.howstuffworks.com/cell-phone.htm.

other wireless devices move in an invisible electric field from an antenna to a receiver. To reach your phone or iPad, for example, this invisible field forms electromagnetic radiation (EMR) that travels through air, trees, buildings, cars, and people.

When a wave oscillates very frequently, like in a microwave, its wave is very short. When a wave oscillates less frequently and more slowly (think of the ocean), its frequency (hertz) will be much lower and its wavelength longer.

A mobile phone's emissions will therefore affect areas nearest to it—like your brain—while you hold it to your head, or, if you keep the phone in your breast pocket, your heart. At lower frequencies near 70 MHz, emissions offer whole-body exposure.

Analog and Digital Signals

Analog signals exist in nature. *Digital* signals do not. Analog signals operate in a wave or at an amplitude that changes slowly and continuously. They are well characterized by a smooth frequency spectrum.

Digital signals are made up of sharp transitions, usually called a pulse in a field or an amplitude. Digital signals usually operate at low amplitudes, but they generate more RF noise in a more complicated, choppy RF spectrum. Depending on the speed and sharpness of its pulse, a digital signal may generate a broader frequency spectrum. This creates more noise for more frequencies and interferes with more equipment.

Near digital devices such as a "smart" utility meter, a cellular antenna, or computer, an AM radio tuned between stations will pick up interference that sounds like buzzing. While engineers recognize that such interference can harm the operation of other electronic devices, few have considered such interference's effects on living creatures.

Pulse and Modulation: Signals Not Found in Nature

Information can be encoded by *modulating* and *pulsing* an electromagnetic signal. There are many kinds of modulation, the manipulation of waves (see the glossary). Modulations are continuous changes. Pulses occur in a pattern of sharp, sudden changes. Individual patterns contain packets of data, not single bits.

AM radio uses *amplitude modulation*: it operates at a single frequency that does not change with time—but the amplitude does.

FM radio is *frequency modulated*, which means it varies the frequency within the band, a larger spectrum than AM radio uses.

Digital or pulsed modulation methods require even wider pieces of the frequency spectrum. Digital or pulsed modulation allows videos and voice and general data to be transmitted with higher quality.

Pulse modulated RF signals are not found in nature. Exposure to these signals increases opportunities for biological (health) effects.[9] Recent studies of modulated RF signals report changes in human cognition, reaction time, brainwave activity, sleep disruptionand immune function.[10]

Electromagnetic Radiation

When electric or magnetic fields change in time, electrical charges respond by accelerating or decelerating and releasing energy into space. This energy release or emission is called electromagnetic radiation (EMR). EMR carries energy that (except for visible light) is usually invisible and that can move through

9 C. Blackman, "Cell phone radiation: Evidence from ELF and RF studies supporting more inclusive risk identification and assessment," *Pathophysiology* vol. 16 (2009): 205–216.

10 Ibid.

space and penetrate most non-metal objects. Mobile phones use EMR to create an invisible wave that can carry your voice or other data. Microwave ovens use EMR to heat food. Whenever moisture is present, such as when EMR passes through a person, some radiation is absorbed.

The Function of an Antenna in Wireless Communications

When EMR encounters an antenna, it generates currents that are measured (demodulated) by a receiver and turned into sound or patterns for television pictures or computer communication. Any conductive object, hence any piece of metal, can serve as an antenna—though many factors, such as size, shape, and orientation determine an antenna's efficiency. A metallic tooth filling can act like an antenna. The electrochemical corrosion of the filling can demodulate a radio signal and act like a receiver.

"Smart" Meters: Transmitting, Digital Utility Meters

A "smart" meter tracks the use of electricity, natural gas, or water. While SmartMeter is a trademarked, industry name that refers to one brand of meter, "smart" meter (no upper case) is the generic term for all new digital meters. Most transmit signals in the microwave range. Some are not transmitting. Some transmitting meters are called "AMR" (automated meter reading) meters. Typically, the meter's face will show a digital display of numbers (like a digital watch), not a dial with a clock-like face. Note: some meters with clock-like faces have a transmitting chip behind their face.

AMI (advanced metering infrastructure) meters are yet another kind of transmitting meter. AMIs provide utility companies with two-way communication. Besides sending your utility company information about your usage, AMIs allow the company to turn off your power remotely or reprogram the meter to communicate with your appliances and your home wireless system.

Around the U.S. and the world, utility companies use government subsidies to replace traditional, analog meters on homes and businesses, supposedly because the "smart" meters' tracking abilities can encourage consumers to conserve energy. "Smart" meters allow utility companies to charge ratepayers by their time-of-use. Here, the aim is for households to use less energy during business hours, to smooth out the peaks and valleys of power consumption and increase the grid's efficiency.[11]

Because every household typically receives three utilities (electricity, gas, and water), and each utility requires a meter on each house, apartment, school, office, hospital, and public building, "smart" meters might be the country's (and the world's) largest deployment of transmitting antennas.

"Smart" meters can use broadband over power lines (BPL), fiber optics, telephone lines or wireless radio, or cellular technology to report detailed information about how much and when you use different "smart enabled" appliances and energy back to the utility company.

"Smart" meters emit pulsed signals or microbursts in the microwave range. Meters using BPL put radio frequency radiation on the power lines. Others transmit in 900 MHz (for the carrier wave) and all use the 2.4 GHz band simultaneously.[12] All creatures within range of these "smart" meters are exposed to involuntary microwave radiation.

Some transmitting meters emit signals once each month or once a day. Some emit signals every fifteen seconds.

✿

Cindy Sage and James J. Biergiel, EMF electrical consultants: *Typical gauge electrical wiring that provides electricity to*

11 K. R. Foster, "A World awash with wireless devices," *IEEE Microwave Magazine*, March, 2013.

12 *SmartMeters: Architecture, Health Effects, Measurement and Mitigation*, a power point presentation by Tom Wilson, BSEE, 2011.

buildings (60 Hz power) is not constructed or intended to carry high frequency harmonics. But the exponential increase in use of appliances, variable speed motors, office and computer equipment and wireless technologies has greatly increased these harmonics in community electrical grids and the buildings they serve with electricity. Harmonics are frequencies higher than 60 Hz that carry more energy and ride on the electrical wiring in bursts. Radio frequency (RF) is an unintentional by-product on the electrical wiring.

Such RF may contribute to electrical fires where there is a weak spot (older wiring, undersized neutrals for the electrical load, poor grounding, use of aluminum conductors, etc.). The use of "smart" meters will place an entirely new and significantly increased burden on existing electrical wiring because of the very short, very high-intensity wireless emissions (radio frequency bursts) that these meters produce to signal the utility about energy usage.

Broadband over Power Lines (BPL)

With BPL, a modem takes its signal from an electric socket, rather than from a phone jack. This allows high-speed Internet access (operating between one and 80 MHz) anywhere with electricity by sending high-frequency electric signals for Internet data on the same power lines that provide low-frequency (60 Hz) power for normal electricity. BPL can send signals four times further than a typical Wi-Fi router.

Unlike cabled modems, BPL provides no shielding. The power lines act as an antenna that wraps around your neighborhood. If your only goal is fast Internet access everywhere, BPL is wonderful. Unfortunately, BPL creates frequency fields in the megahertz range and significant electrical transient noise on power lines. At these high frequencies, most households' wiring will expose inhabitants to RF electric and magnetic fields.

Fiber Optics

Fiber optics transmit data by pulsing signals on a light wave through a single hair-like fiber of glass or plastic. With this technology, each residence, school, and business can access the Internet, much like most of us have landline service available. Initially, fiber optics are expensive to install. Long-term, they provide the fastest, safest, most energy-efficient, and most secure service. They can be installed to produce no radiated emissions.

Many fiber optics systems terminate into a "cable box." This box may provide for wired or wireless services—including Ethernet, Wi-Fi, TV, and telephone. The Ethernet provides a wired connection to laptop or desktop computers, and requires no radio transmitters. Wireless services (Wi-Fi, some TV and some telephones) require a radio transmitter that continuously emits microwaves.

Telecommunications services can be delivered through fiber optics without transmitters. However, in some areas where fiber optics have been installed, residents do not have the option of turning off their wireless router. Pregnant women, infants, children, people with medical implants and those with compromised health may be especially vulnerable.

Like so many other new technologies, implementing fiber optics safely requires more testing and protective regulation.

Our New Electromagnetic Environment

We now live in an electromagnetic environment that is complex beyond human control. Since the 1930s, the FCC has allowed manufacturers to market new devices and services as long as they do not interfere with existing radio, TV, or Internet broadcasts. Inventors have not been required to prove that their devices do not cause biological harm.

Let's look at the question: *how do magnetic fields, electronics and wireless devices affect human health?*

6

Health Effects of Exposure to Magnetic and Radio-Frequency Fields

It is no measure of health to be well adjusted to a profoundly sick society.

Krishnamurti

Figure this: every organ in the human body gets information about how to function from electrical or electrochemical signals. The brain, heart, blood, muscles, nerves, kidneys, and digestive organs each has its own dominant frequency;[1] and organs communicate to each other by electromagnetic signals. An adult heart, beating seventy times per minute, has a hertz rate of 1.17.[2] A baby's heart, beating 120 times per minute, has a hertz rate of two.[3] The nervous system operates at multiple frequencies. Brainwaves operate mostly between 2 Hz and 20 Hz; the brain rests at about 10 Hz.[4]

---

1 J. Oschman, *Energy Medicine*, London: Churchill Livingstone, 2000.

2 *The New Book of Popular Science*, Grolier, 1996; also F. Magill, *Magill's Survey of Science*, Hackensack, NJ: Salem Press, 1991.

3 G. Lietz and Anne White, *Secrets of the Heart and Blood*, Durham, UK: Gerrard, 1965.

4 J. Oschman, *Energy Medicine*.

To function, our bodies also receive cues from hormones, chemistry, and the Earth's electromagnetic fields.[5] We rarely perceive these cues consciously. Bees, birds, cows, fish, plants, and trees—indeed all living creatures—function by using internal electromagnetic signals and by receiving external ones.

ꕥ

Paul Martinez, 24, New York: *In school, I learned that the mind is most restful when it cycles about ten times per second. Most of the Earth's electromagnetic fields vibrate under 10 Hz. These fields are called the Schumann Resonances. So: a restful mind vibrates in sync with the Earth. But our buildings are wired for 60 Hz, and we're surrounded by devices that commonly vibrate millions and billions of times per second. How do I deal with this if my goal is a restful mind?*

We all know that some people smoke several packs of cigarettes every day and never get sick. Some people get lung cancer or other diseases from second-hand smoke. Likewise, every person arrives at the threshold of exposure to magnetic fields and radio-frequency fields uniquely. People who live, study, and/or work within buildings with wiring errors; near transformers, transmission lines, cellular antennas, transmitting utility meters; and who use mobile phones and Wi-Fi may be exposed to more radiation than people who have correctly wired homes far from transformers, use only corded phones, have no Wi-Fi, and live and work more than a mile from an antenna in buildings that have no transmitting utility meters.

In reality, most of us are probably exposed to magnetic fields, since more than fifty percent of homes in the U.S. have wiring errors.

---

5 R. Becker, MD, *The Body Electric: Electromagnetism and the Foundation of Life,* New York: William Morrow, 1985.

As for radiation from wireless technologies, from 2005 to 2007, the number of cell phone subscribers in the U.S. increased from 13% to 84% of our population. In 2010, more than 91% of our country's 308 million people had cell phones.[6] Worldwide, the vast majority of our planet's seven billion people now have mobile service. By 2016, Cisco estimates that 1.2 million minutes of video will be streamed or downloaded every second.[7] The cellular antennas that transmit signals for wireless devices are now ubiquitous, as are transmitting utility meters.

So what are the biological effects of exposure to electrosmog?

Part One:
Human Health, Magnetic Fields and Stray Voltage

In the 1970s, Colorado epidemiologist Nancy Wertheimer began reporting cancer clusters and other health problems caused by exposure to magnetic fields. Around the same time, epidemiologist Samuel Milham, MD observed a connection between electrification and "diseases of civilization," including cancer, cardiovascular disease, diabetes, suicide, and Alzheimer's.[8] Dr. Milham also identified that electrical workers, electricians, radio and power station operators, and people who work in the aluminum industry—all of whom are exposed to strong magnetic fields—have an elevated risk of leukemia.[9] Teachers who work in classrooms with high

6 See www.ctia.org/advocacy/research/index.cfm/AID/10323.

7 *Washington Post*, 11-29-2012, "Web video leaves deaf out of loop."

8 S. Milham, MD, MPH, *Dirty Electricity*, iUniverse.com, 2010.

9 "Exposures to Extra Low Frequency EMFs in Occupations with Elevated Leukemia Rates," *Applied Industrial Hygiene* vol. 3, no. 6 (1988): 189–193.

frequency voltage transients on the wires have an increased risk of a variety of cancers.[10]

A study at California's Kaiser Permanente Hospital showed that women who used video display terminals (VDTs) more than twenty hours per week had twice the number of miscarriages as women who did not use VDTs, and their offspring had increased birth defects.[11]

Nancy Wertheimer and Ed Leeper also found that when pregnant women used electric blankets and waterbeds, they had a higher incidence of miscarriages. The highest risks occurred in winter, when electric blanket use is greater.[12]

A study of suicidal deaths between 1969 and 1976 in the West Midlands, England, published in the August, 1981 issue of *Health Physics* by F. Stephen Perry and colleagues, "Environmental Power-Frequency Magnetic Fields and Suicide," showed that "significantly more suicides occurred at locations of high magnetic field strength."

According to longtime watchdog *Microwave News*, "strong epidemiological evidence" shows that exposure to magnetic fields is a risk factor for Alzheimer's. Seamstresses who use industrial sewing machines are particularly vulnerable. A meta-analysis of fourteen occupational studies showed that exposure to EMFs on the job doubled the risk of developing Alzheimer's. People living within fifty meters of a high-voltage power line were more likely to die with Alzheimer's. The longer they lived

10 S. Milham and L. L. Morgan, "A new electromagnetic exposure metric: High frequency voltage transients associated with increased cancer incidence in teachers in a California school," *American Journal of Industrial Medicine*, vol. 51 (2008): 579–586.

11 M. K. Goldhaber, *American Journal of Industrial Medicine,* vol. 25 (1988): 150–155.

12 N. Wertheimer and E. Leeper, "Possible effects of electric blankets and heated waterbeds on fetal development," *Bioelectromagnetics* vol. 7 (1986): 13–22.

near a 220 to 380 kV power line, the greater the risk: after fifteen years, the odds of dying with Alzheimer's were double the expected rate.[13]

Safety Standards for Magnetic Fields

According to our federal Occupational Safety and Hazard Administration (OSHA) standards (determined by engineers), magnetic fields above one gauss—1000 mG—are dangerous.

Those who study health have made other conclusions. Because of the possible link between childhood leukemia and *in utero* exposure to ELFs, *The BioInitiative 2012 Report* (a compilation of 1,800 studies about the biological effects of electromagnetic fields and radio frequency radiation, edited by Cindy Sage, MA and David O. Carpenter, MD) recommends a 1.0 mG limit for existing habitable space for children and/or pregnant women, *To be clear, the BioInitiative Group recommends 1/1000th of what OSHA allows.*

The Seletun Statement, made by an international, scientific panel that met in Seletun, Norway in 2009, also recommends a limit of 1.0 mG exposure "for all new installations based on findings of risk for leukemia, brain tumours, Alzheimer's, ALS, sperm damage, and DNA strand breaks."

The Institute for Building Biology (which provides environmental consulting primarily in Europe and the U.S.) considers readings below 0.2 mG of "no concern." Readings between 0.2 and 1.0 mG are of "slight concern." Readings between 1.0 and 5.0 mG are of "severe concern." Readings above 5.0 mG are of "extreme concern."[14]

ꕥ

13 L. Slesin, "Power-line EMFs: New focus on Alzheimer's disease," *Microwave News*, 11-17-2008.

14 International Institute for Building-Biology and Ecology, *Electromagnetic Radiation Seminar Manual,* 212, 2011.

Lydia Shuster, 74, Washington: *I've enjoyed extremely good health all of my life. In 1985, I moved into a ground level apartment near Seattle. Starting in 2009, I gradually noticed a variety of ailments: about fifteen minutes after I went to bed, my upper legs would itch. Then, when I scratched, small bumps would appear. The rash would be gone by morning, but I woke up feeling like I hadn't rested, with debilitating, achy joints. I had difficulty concentrating. My hair started falling out. I moved in fuzzy, slow motion.*

When I left my condo for a couple of hours or more, my symptoms seemed to clear considerably. If I went out of town, within twelve hours, all of the symptoms would be gone. So I began to think that something in my condo was making me sick. I knew that several of the buildings in my association had severe mold issues.

In 2012, I hired a building biology consultant. She found mold in my shower stall. Then, with her gauss meter, she measured the magnetic fields in and around my condo. My bedroom measured 1.7 mG. At the transformer about thirty feet from me (across a parking lot), the reading showed 7 mG. The consultant found both of these readings alarming, since magnetic fields can harm health.

I moved out of my bedroom and began sleeping on my couch, where the gauss meter showed 1.2 mG. After a few weeks, I no longer had a rash. My joints improved by 80%. I still experience tiredness.

Following the building biologist's suggestion, I also quit using my cordless phone. Then, once, I used it for a long call. I had shooting pains and a headache for two days. So that gave me a good lesson. I put the cordless phone away.

It took me two months to convince my electric company to send an engineer to assess the situation. At my bedroom window, his gauss meter read 1.8 mG to 2.4 mG. My microwave oven, which is built into a wall in my very small kitchen so that I can't unplug it, showed 54 mG while running, Turned off, it measured 43 mG. After the engineer got these readings, he would not stay in my kitchen. When he left, I shut off the wires that go to the microwave at my circuit breaker panel.

Yet later, a contractor found a leak and mold in my crawl space. Then, I discovered www.emf-portal.de, which posts studies about the relationship between mold and magnetic fields.

Meanwhile, the utility company emailed me that the magnetic fields in my condo are well within government standards, and that no further investigation is warranted.

I have friends reporting brain tumors and severe heart problems. We all need to pay attention and decrease our use of radiation-emitting devices.

Stray Voltage and Health

Stray voltage, electricity that travels on the ground, can also harm health. It occurs when the neutral wire that returns current to its source (the substation) is not sufficient. In March, 2013, a woman won a four million dollar lawsuit against Southern California Edison because she repeatedly got shocked from stray voltage that electrified her shower head.[15] Dogs and cows (who do not cover their soles with rubber) have been electrocuted by stray voltage.[16]

15 B. Greenfield, "Woman Shocked in Shower Wins $4 Million Lawsuit: Is Your Shower Safe?" *Shine*, 3-21-2013.

16 Dr. Magda Havas, speaking in Feb. 2013 in a public forum sponsored by the Perth County Federation of Agriculture in Listowel, Ontario; reported by Bob Reid in *Ontario Farmer*.

Part Two:
Human Health and Wireless Devices

David O. Carpenter, MD, and Cindy Sage, MA, *BioInitiative 2012 Report,* Section 24: *Bioeffects are clearly established and occur at very low levels of exposure to electromagnetic fields and radio frequency radiation. Bioeffects can occur in the first few minutes at levels associated with cell and cordless phone use. Bioeffects can also occur from just minutes of exposure to cellular base antennas, Wi-Fi and wireless utility "smart" meters that produce whole-body exposure. Chronic base station level exposures can result in illness. Many of these bioeffects can reasonably be expected to result in adverse health effects if the exposures are prolonged or chronic. This is because they interfere with normal body processes (disrupt homeostasis), prevent the body from healing damaged DNA, produce immune system imbalances, metabolic disruption and lower resistance to disease across multiple pathways.*

The Health Effects of Ionizing and Non-Ionizing Radiation

Before I report how wireless devices affect health, let me spell out different perspectives on the health effects of ionizing and non-ionizing radiation. (As explained in the previous chapter, radio frequency fields, including microwaves used by wireless devices, are non-ionizing.)

Scientists agree that the health effects of ionizing radiation are cumulative, and that these effects can harm and kill. For example, brief exposure to (ionizing) ultra violet light can cause an immediate sunburn. With enough exposure, a person might get cataracts or skin cancer.

Since non-ionizing radiation (emitted by radio, TV, and Internet broadcasts and mobile phones) usually does not heat tissue immediately, scientists disagree about whether or not it impacts health. However, in a microwave oven, non-ionizing radiation causes water molecules to rotate rapidly in a frictional medium and produce heat. If the temperature rises high or long enough, and if its amplitude is strong enough, then non-ionizing radiation can cause tissue damage immediately.

The human body is two thirds water. Does cumulative exposure to non-ionizing radiation affect health? This is a controversy. Whether or not tissue is heated, many other biological effects occur; but not all scientists recognize non-ionizing radiation's non-thermal effects. All would recognize ionizing radiation's non-thermal effects.

Thermal and Non-Thermal Effects

Again, the FCC has so far determined the safety of wireless devices solely by their immediate *thermal* effects: when a six-foot-two mannequin weighing more than two hundred pounds (his head filled with fluid) used a cell phone for six minutes and his temperature did not change more than one degree Celsius, the FCC determined that cell phones are safe.[17]

Meanwhile, many scientists have found numerous *non-thermal,* biological effects from using mobile phones:

- After twenty minutes of use, double-strands of DNA break into fragments. If the body's repair systems can't keep up with these breaks, cancer and birth defects can result.[18]
- Cancer rates increase, especially when people begin using mobile phones as children and when anyone uses one for thirty minutes or more per day. The risk of tumors also

17 D. Davis, *Disconnect: The Truth about Cell Phone Radiation, What the Industry Is Doing to Hide It, and How to Protect Your Family,* New York: Dutton, 2010.

18 A. Campisi et al, "Reactive oxygen species levels and DNA fragmentation on astrocytes in primary culture after acute exposure to low intensity microwave electromagnetic field," *Neuroscience Letters*, vol. 473 (2010): 52–55, .

increases significantly with over ten years of cell phone use.[19]

- After two hours of use, the blood–brain barrier begins to leak, allowing neurotoxins in food, air, or water to affect the brain and nerves, eventually leading to brain cell death.[20]
- For digital cell phone users who began using a cell phone as teenagers or younger, the increased risk of brain cancer is 420%.[21]
- Prenatal exposure to cell phones results in emotional and hyperactive problems in children around the time they reach school age.[22]
- Exposure to electromagnetic fields activates voltage-gated calcium channels. This leads to increased calcium levels within cells, which leads to the production of a series of compounds including peroxynitrite. Peroxynitrite is at the root

---

19 E. Cardis et al, "Brain tumor risk in relation to mobile telephone use: Results of the Interphone International Case Controlled Study," *International Journal of Epidemiology*, vol. 39, no. 3 (2010): 675–694; L. Hardell et al, "Epidemiological evidence for an association between use of wireless phones and tumor diseases," *Pathophysiology*, Aug. 2009, vol. 16., (2–3), 113–122; L. Hardell et al, "Tumor risk associated with use of cellular telephones or cordless desktop telephones, *World Journal of Surgical Oncology*, vol. 4, no. 74 (2006); L. Hardell et al, "Long-term use of cellular phones and brain tumors; increased risk associated with use for >or = 10 years, *Occupational and Environmental Medicine*, vol. 64 (2007): 626–632; Ö. Hallberg et al, "The potential impact of mobile phone use on trends in brain and CNS tumors," *Journal of Neurology and Neurophysiology*, Dec. 2011.

20 L. G. Salford et al, "Nerve cell damage in mammalian brain after exposure to microwaves from GSM mobile phones," *Environmental Health Perspectives*, vol. 111, no. 7, (2003).

21 L. Hardell and M. Carlberg, "Mobile phones, cordless phones and the risk for brain tumors," *International Journal of Oncology*, vol. 35 (2009): 5–17.

22 H. Divan et al, "Prenatal and postnatal exposure to cell phone use and behavioral problems in children," *Epidemiology*, vol. 19, no. 4 (2008).

of most inflammatory diseases, including neurodegenerative and cardiovascular diseases, migraines, and allergies.[23]

ꕤ

Andrew Goldsworthy, PhD, professor emeritus of biology at London's Imperial College: *Is damage done by digital telecommunications due only to heating? Is it due to the electrical effect that their pulsating signals have on live tissue? The human body can act as an antenna, and signals from electronics and wireless devices can make electric currents flow through the body with the pulsations. This destabilizes the delicate membranes that surround each cell, which constitutes biological harmful interference: normal operation of cells and normal communication between cells are disrupted.*

Cell membranes are just two molecules thick. They are liquid crystals, made largely of negatively charged molecules that repel each other. They are stabilized by divalent positive ions (mostly calcium) that sit between them by mutual attraction and hold them together like mortar holds together the bricks in a wall.

In 1975, Suzanne Bawin and her coworkers showed us that modulated radio frequency electromagnetic radiation that is far too weak to heat tissue significantly can remove calcium ions (positively charged calcium ions) from cell membranes in the brain.[24] Actually, weak electromagnetic fields can have a greater effect than strong ones; prolonged exposure to weak radio frequency fields (where cells are maintained in the unstable condition for longer) is potentially

---

23 M. Pall, "Electromagnetic fields act via activation of voltage-gated calcium channels to produce beneficial or adverse effects," *Journal of Cellular and Molecular Medicine*, 6-26-2013.

24 S. M. Bawin et al, "Effects of modulated VHF fields on the central nervous system," *Academy of Science,* 247: 74–81.

more damaging than relatively brief exposure to much stronger fields.[25]

The loss of calcium is important, because calcium ions bind to and stabilize the cell's negatively charged membranes. Loss of just some of these calcium ions destabilizes the membrane and makes it more inclined to leak, which can have serious metabolic consequences.

For example, membrane leakage affects our neurons. Neurons transmit information between each other by chemical neurotransmitters that pass across the synapses where they make contact. Normally, neurotransmitters are triggered to release their neurotransmitters by a brief pulse of calcium entering the cell. If the membrane is leaky due to electromagnetic exposure, it will already have a high internal concentration of calcium. This puts the cells into hair-trigger mode: they are more likely to release neurotransmitters, and the brain as a whole may become hyperactive.[26] *The brain may become overloaded, leading to a loss of concentration, Attention Deficit Hyperactive Disorder (ADHD), damage to DNA due to the release of reactive oxygen species from mitochondria, and digestive enzymes from lysosomes. Such DNA damage can cause a loss of fertility and an increased risk of getting cancer.*

Membrane leakage can also open the blood–brain barrier, leading to Alzheimer's and early dementia. Damage to similar barriers that protect all of our body surfaces from foreign

---

25 A. Goldsworthy, electromagnetichealth.org/wp-content/uploads/2010/04/why_vodafone_should_not_increase2.pdf 2010.

26 R. C. Beason and P. Semm, "Responses of neurons to an amplitude modulated microwave stimulus," *Neuroscience Letters,* vol. 333 (2002): 175–178; J. F. Krey and R. E. Dolmetsch, "Molecular mechanisms of autism: A possible role for Ca2+ signaling," *Current Opinion in Neurobiology,* vol. 17 (2007): 12–119; N. D. Volkow et al, , "Effects of Cell Phone Radio frequency Signal Exposure on Brain Glucose Metabolism," *Journal of the American Medical Association,* vol. 305 no. 8 (2011): 808–813. doi: 10.1001/jama.2011.186.

chemicals can exacerbate a variety of illnesses, including asthma, allergies, and auto-immune disorders such as multiple sclerosis.[27]

SAR: A Measure of Radiation Absorbed by Body Tissue

The amount of radiation that tissue absorbs while exposed to a mobile device is called the device's Specific Absorption Rate (SAR). SAR measures the ratio of power to weight (watt/kilogram) at a given frequency above 100 kHz for a given period of time. A SAR is useful in a controlled laboratory that measures single-source, single-frequency exposures on mannequins. Beyond the lab, where isolation of a single frequency is likely impossible, a true SAR may not be obtainable.

A SAR is most relevant for quantifying radiation exposure from devices that are used near the body. Before 1996, our federal government provided no regulation of mobile devices held near your body. Starting in 1996, the FCC allowed a SAR of 1.6 W/kg or less for 1 gram of tissue. (1 g of body tissue is defined as tissue volume in the shape of a cube.)

In August, 2013, the FCC revised its SAR standards. Based on recommendations from the Institute of Electrical and Electronics Engineers (IEEE), the new standards reclassify the pinna (the outer part of the ear) as an extremity—the same as the feet, ankles, hands, and wrists. Extremities are permitted a SAR of 4.0 W/kg for any 10 g of tissue more than 30 minutes.

In 2004, electrical engineers Dr. Om Gandhi and Dr. Gang King voiced their concerns about this (then proposed) revision in the IEEE's peer-reviewed journal, *Transactions on Microwave Theory and Techniques*. They wrote that treating the pinna as

27 Find more at hese-project.org/hese-uk/en/papers/cell_phone_and_cell.pdf and at bioinitiative.org. Dr. Martin Pall's paper, "Electromagnetic fields act via activation of voltage-gated calcium channels to produce beneficial or adverse effects," analyzes 24 studies in *Journal of Cellular and Molecular Medicine*, 6-26-2013.

an extremity would allow cell phone radiation at levels that are eight to sixteen times higher than levels allowed by the regulations established in 1996. The pinna is close to the brain. In fact, it acts as a conduit for cell phone radiation into the head. Thus, allowing 4.0 W/kg for any 10 grams of tissue will result in considerably higher cell phone radiated power levels. 4.0 W/kg is up to two times higher than levels permitted under international ICNIRP guidelines followed in over thirty countries.

Further, children have thinner skulls than adults. Scientists from the U.S., Japan, Spain, Brazil, France, and Switzerland[28] have shown in peer-reviewed journals that when children use cell phones, they absorb about two times as much radiation as adults do.

In 2013, typical mobile phones had a SAR of 1.6 W/kg. With the FCC's reclassifying the pinna of the ear as an extremity, presumably, mobile devices could have a SAR of 4.0 W/kg.

---

28 O. P. Gandhi et al, "Electromagnetic absorption in the human head and neck for mobile telephones at 835 and 1,900 MHz," IEEE, *Transactions on Microwave Theory and Techniques*, vol. 44 (1996): 1,884–1,892; O. P. Gandhi and G. Kang, "Some present problems and a proposed experimental phantom for SAR compliance testing of cellular telephones at 835 and 1,900 MHz," *Physics in Medicine and Biology*, vol. 47 (2002): 1,501–1,518; J. Wang and O. Fujiwara, "Comparison and evaluation of electromagnetic absorption characteristics in realistic human head models of adults and children for 900 MHz mobile telephones," IEEE *Transactions on Microwave Theory and Techniques*, vol. 51 (2003): 966–971; M. Martinez-Burdalo et al, "Comparison of FDTD-calculated specific absorption rate in adults and children when using a mobile phone at 900 and 1,800 MHz," *Physics in Medicine and Biology,* vol. 49 (2004): 345–354; A. De Salles et al, "Electromagnetic absorption in the head of adults and children due to mobile phone operation close to the head," *Electromagnetic Biology and Medicine*, vol. 25 (2006): 349–360; J. Wiart et al, "Analysis of RF exposure in the head tissues of children and adults," *Physics in Medicine and Biology*, vol. 53 (2008): 3681–3695; N. Kuster et al, "Past, present and future research on the exposure of children," *Foundation for Research on Information Technology in Society, Foundation Internal Report*, 2009.

No agency regulates the effects of a cell phone's SAR on children.

Also note that some manufacturers of implanted medical devices (i.e., insulin pumps, cardiac pacemakers, and deep brain stimulators) warn users against an exposure greater than 0.1 W/kg for fifteen minutes.[29] Anyone with "smart" meters, Wi-Fi, broadband over power lines, cellular antennas, or mobile phone users in their area may find it impossible to limit exposure to this level.

How Do SAR Levels below 1.6W/Kg Affect Long-Term Health?

Rat studies have shown reduced memory (immediately) and early dementia (long-term) with exposure below 0.6 W/kg.[30] With exposures below 1.2 W/kg, single and double strand DNA breaks result immediately; long-term, brain tumors[31] and dementia result.[32] Early dementia, ALS, Parkinson's, and other neurological diseases occur long-term with exposure to SAR levels below 0.12 W/kg.[33] Another study found, at exposures below .12 W/kg, that normal DNA repair is impaired, the immune system

29 See www.MRIsafety.com.

30 H. Lai et al, "Microwave irradiation affects radial-arm maze performance in the rat," *Bioelectromagnetics*, vol. 15, no. 2 (1994): 95–104.

31 H. Lai and N. Singh, "Single- and double-strand DNA breaks in rat brain cells after acute exposure to radio-frequency electromagnetic radiation," *International Journal of Radiation Biology,* vol. 69, no. 4 (1996): 513–21; E. Diem et al, "Non-thermal DNA breakage by mobile phone radiation (1,800 MHz) in human fibroblasts and in transformed GFSH-R17 rat granulosa cells in vitro," *Mutation Research,* vol. 583, no. 2 (2005):178–83.

32 B. Wang and H. Lai, "Acute exposure to pulsed 2,450 MHz microwaves affects water-maze performance of rats," *Bioelectromagnetics*, vol. 21, no. 1 (2000): 52–56.

33 J. Eberhardt et al, "Blood–brain barrier permeability and nerve cell damage in rat brain 14 and 28 days after exposure to microwaves from GSM mobile phones," *Electromagnetic Biology and Medicine*, vol. 27, no. 3 (2008): 215–29.

malfunctions, and birth defects occur.[34] Exposed to cell-phone radiation at an early age at SAR levels between .016 W/kg and 2.0 W/kg, rats developed learning problems, ADD/ADHD, early dementia, Parkinson's, ALS, and other neurological diseases.[35]

ꕤ

Gary Olhoeft, PhD: *I have Parkinson's disease. In 2009, I had a deep brain stimulator (DBS) implanted in my brain. It completely replaces the pharmaceuticals I took for fifteen years, which caused increasingly unpleasant side effects. My Medtronics manual says that a cell phone must be at least 20 inches away from me with a SAR of no more than 1.8. Held near my head, the phone's SAR can't be more than 0.25 for 15 minutes. Otherwise, according to Medtronics, it will cause dangerous heating of my implant. If the implant gets too hot, it will malfunction, my brain could be injured, or I could die.*

Second-hand SAR, like second-hand cigarette smoke, occurs from exposure to EMR sources without benefit—like when being near someone using a mobile phone or Wi-Fi. The effects of second-hand SAR on health (including babies exposed in utero to their mothers' mobile phones and laptops, children and people with medical implants) have not been studied.

While emissions from a cell phone may primarily affect the area nearest the phone (i.e., the brain, throat, heart, abdomen, or genitals), emissions from Wi-Fi and/or 4G reach the whole body.

To learn the SAR for a specific mobile device, find its FCC ID number on its case or after removing the battery pack. Then,

---

34 I. Pavacic et al, "In vitro testing of cellular response to ultra high frequency electromagnetic field radiation," *Toxicology in Vitro,* no. 5, (2008): 1,344–1,348.

35 O. Bas et al, "900 MHz electromagnetic field exposure affects qualitative and quantitative features of hippocampal pyramidal cells in the adult female rat," *Brain Research*, vol. 1,265 (04-10-2009): 178–185.

go to equipmentauthorization.gov; click on "FCC ID Search." Enter the ID's first three characters in "Grantee Code," and the remaining characters under "Equipment Product Code." Then, click on "Start Search" and "Display Grant."

A Historical Context for the Biological Effects of RF Signals

In 1953, the Soviets installed a wireless system that radiated the American embassy in Moscow, a system that continued until the mid-seventies. (The Soviets' intention for this installation remains controversial.) Because they were exposed to radio frequency radiation, many of the workers, including ambassadors, got leukemia and other diseases. The "low-level" of radiation that employees were exposed to was remarkably similar to exposures people now experience when they live near cellular antennas.

Soviet medical researchers first identified a syndrome they called microwave sickness, now called electro-hypersensitivity (EHS). The Soviets found that exposure to RF radiation can develop into tumors, blood changes, reproductive and cardiovascular abnormalities, depression, and other problems.[36]

The U.S. Senate also studied the effects of low-level radiation emitted by the Soviets on personnel who worked at the U.S. Embassy.[37] The U.S. Senate's Lilienfield Study found eczema, psoriasis, allergic and inflammatory reactions; neurological and reproductive problems; an increase of tumors (malignant in women, benign in men); blood abnormalities; and effects on mood and well-being including irritability, depression, loss of appetite, concentration, and eye problems. These symptoms are nearly

36 M. S. Tolgskaya and A. V. Gordon, "Pathological effects of radio waves," Soviet Science Consultants Bureau, New York, 1973 133–137.

37 U.S. Senate, 1979. "Microwave radiation of the U.S. Embassy in Moscow," Committee on Commerce, Science and Transportation, 90th Congress, 1st session, April 1979, 1–23.

identical to those reported by people with EHS and in studies of communities exposed to radiation from digital signals.[38]

EHS symptoms can also include disturbed sleep, rashes, facial flushing, heart arrhythmia, muscle spasms, memory loss, sinusitis, deteriorating vision, seizures, paralysis, tinnitus, elevated blood sugar levels, stroke, nosebleeds, and digestive problems.

Dietrich Klinghardt, MD has explored the relationship between EHS and Lyme disease (klinghardtacademy.com).

Recently, the California Department of Health found that three percent of Californians (770,000 people) believe they have some form of EHS or radio-frequency sickness. Five percent of Swiss people experience RF Sickness.[39] Up to 9% of Germany's 2004 population, and 13.3% of Taiwan's 2010 population[40] experience electro-hypersensitivity.

If three percent of the U.S. population has RF Sickness, that's more than nine million people.

Why do some people experience RF Sickness and others—even in the same household or workplace—not experience it? Let's answer this question with two more: Why do some people

38 R. Santini et al, "Enquete sur la sante de riverains de stations relais de telephonie mobile: Incidences de la distance et du sexe. *Pathologie Biologie,* vol. 50 (2002): 369–373, doi.10.1016/50369-8114(02)00311–5; G. Abdel-Rassoul et al, "Neurobehavioral effects among inhabitants around mobile phone base stations," *Neurotoxicology,* vol. 22, no. 2 (2007): 434–440, doi.10.1016/j.neuro.2006.07.012; A. E. Navarro et al, "The microwave syndrome: a preliminary study in Spain, *Electromagnetic Biology and Medicine*, vol. 22, nos. 2–3 (2003): 161–169, doi;10.1081/JBC-120024625; B. Levitt and H. Lai, "Biological effects from exposure to electromagnetic radiation emitted by cell tower base stations and other antenna arrays," *Environmental Reviews,* vol. 18 (2010): 369–395.

39 See www.dirtyelectricity.ca/images/Swiss%20EMF%20study.pdf

40 M. Tseng et al, "Prevalence and psychiatric comorbidity of self-reported electromagnetic field sensitivity in Taiwan: a population-based study," *Journal of the Formosan Medical Association,* vol. 110 (2011): 634–641.

smoke two packs of cigarettes every day and keep "healthy?" Why do some people get lung cancer from exposure to secondhand smoke?

ꕥ

Richard Conrad, PhD, biochemist, conradbiologic.com: *Exposure to a new electronic or wireless device, or spending an unusually long time near a device that was previously tolerated can initiate Electro-hypersensitivity. Physical symptoms are then re-triggered by exposure to much lower field levels, levels far below those the FCC considers "safe." Some people are predisposed toward developing EHS because they were exposed earlier to toxins such as pesticides or heavy metals.*

I have talked to numerous scientists, engineers, programmers, financial advisors and realtors who love their work and their computers, but can no longer sit in front of a computer for more than a few minutes without getting debilitating symptoms. They can only drive older cars with early, less powerful computers under the hood. They can't travel into many environments. They are truly disabled.

The World Health Organization on RF Radiation and Health

As I reported in chapter 2, in May 2011, the WHO International Agency for Research on Cancer (IARC) classified radiofrequency radiation as *possibly carcinogenic* to humans, based on an increased risk for glioma, a malignant type of brain cancer (common in the San Diego State cluster), when cell phones are used. IARC has also given this classification to DDT, lead, chloroform, and asbestos.

In a November 2011 lecture at Harvard Law School, Dr. Franz Adlkofer discussed the difficulties that he and other scientists face when presenting research on the carcinogenic effects of electromagnetic fields emitted by cell phones and the institutional corruption that he says obstructs scientists' research. He described the European Union's 2004 REFLEX study,[41] which demonstrated that cell phones that emit RFs below allowed exposure limits display gene-damaging potential. According to Dr. Adlkofer, if IARC had considered studies like REFLEX, it likely would have called cell phone radiation "probably" carcinogenic.

Before 2011, WHO reported that evidence of harm from cell phone use was not convincing. However, this report was authored by Michael Repacholi, an industry consultant who received hundreds of thousands of dollars from corporations with vested interests.[42]

It's also worth noting that Dr. Gro Harlem Brundtland, MD, MPH, who served as Director General of the WHO from 1998 to 2003 (and, earlier, two terms as Norway's Prime Minister), does not allow cell phones in her office. Within four meters of a mobile phone, she gets headaches.[43]

The Interphone Study

To date, Interphone is the largest and longest study to consider the relationship between cell phones and brain tumors. Funded in part by the industry, the average person in the study used a cell phone for four minutes per day. People who used a cell phone for thirty minutes per day over a ten-year period on one side of the head had a 40% increased risk of a brain tumor.

---

41 Risk Evaluation of Potential Environmental Hazards from Low Frequency Electromagnetic Field Exposure Using Sensitive In Vitro Methods.

42 L. Slesin, "It's official: Mike Repacholi is an industry consultant and he's already in hot water," *Microwave News*, 11-13-2006; L. Slesin, "WHO and electric utilities: A partnership on EMFs," *Microwave News*, 10-1-2005.

43 A. Dalsegg, "Mobile phone radiation gives Gro Harlem Brundtland headaches," *Dagbladet*, Oslo, 3-9-2002.

(Today, a half-hour of daily mobile phone use would be considered "light" use; at the time of the study, it was considered "heavy.")

The study did not consider the user's exposure to a phone that is on standby, carried in a pocket or near the head while sleeping. It did not consider the combined risk of exposure from cell phones, cordless phones, Wi-Fi, living near antennas, and/or "smart" meters. It did not consider the risks of cell phone use incurred by pregnant women, infants, children, teens, young adults, or people with medical implants.

"Second-Hand" Exposure To RF Radiation and Health

Robert Kane, Ph.D., electrical engineer, author of *Cellular Telephone Russian Roulette:* *A Historical and Scientific Perspective* **(Vantage Press, 2001):** *Prior to the 1980s, human exposure to radio frequency radiating sources was pretty much restricted to the occasional passing police car, commercial mobile radio, or the ultra low-level RF energies emitted by the sun and a sparse array of remotely located television and radio broadcast antennae. Today, it is virtually impossible to venture into a public place without being battered by unwanted radio frequency radiation from a variety of sources.*

Available research indicates that operation of a nearby portable cellular telephone will expose a non-user to radiation, some of which will be deposited into the non-user's brain at levels higher than necessary to elicit undesirable biological effects, even though the phone may be more than ten feet away from the non-user.

In 1992, Robert Kane sued Motorola, claiming that he developed a brain tumor as a result of testing a prototype antenna for a cell phone while employed by the company. The case was settled as a confidential employer-employee resolution. Dr. Kane died in March, 2005. He was 56.

Alex Richards, tech executive and entrepreneur, 60, California: *I bought my first cell phone in 1990. It felt like a brick. It had a really long antenna that I pulled out for each call, and it cost more than $500. Still, I was ecstatic to own it: my clients could reach me anywhere. Back then, cell phone conversations rarely lasted long, because calls cost a dollar a minute. By 2000, with a lighter phone and a more affordable plan. I spent 2,000 minutes on it each month.*

One day in 2003, waiting in an airport for my luggage, I suddenly felt an electric jolt followed by drilling in the back of my head. I turned around: seven people were using cell phones. I grabbed my bag, left the airport, and the pain went away.

Over the next few years, repeatedly, I would feel drilling—then notice someone nearby on a cell phone. I still had one, but I didn't think it caused me problems. It was analog, not digital; and I seldom used it.

Meanwhile, I focused on my health. For example, I used my landline and got a speakerphone. Once, a client couldn't hear me clearly, so I used my headset. After about a minute and a half, I felt burning in my head that lasted an hour and a half. Later that day, I used the receiver, not the headset, and I felt heat again. So then I learned that I could only use the speakerphone.

I also began to wonder if my cell phone caused me trouble. I didn't use it for a week. Then, the first time I tried it, I felt burning in my head.

In 2006, suddenly, after a vacation, I felt exhausted, and I had drilling in my head again. If I moved from my chair, the drilling stopped. I quit my cell phone entirely that day. I took out our Wi-Fi, cordless phones, wireless printers, fluorescent lights and the electronic garage door opener.

I still felt sick. I started waking in the middle of the night, extremely anxious. I felt like an antenna: I could pick up signals from cordless phones, Wi-Fi, taxi cab and police radios, game stations and cell towers.

My wife doubted my "electro-sensitivity." She figured I had a brain tumor or a psychological issue. So, I went to a neurologist and a neuropsychologist who tested my memory, cognitive abilities and mental health. They also kept a cell phone in the room with its ringer off and told me to raise my hand whenever a call came in. During eight hours of testing, I raised my hand eleven out of thirteen times within seconds of the call. By the test's end, the doctors and my wife no longer doubted my sensitivity. (Apparently, when a call comes in, the cell phone emits microwaves to confirm receipt; some people can sense them.)

I could feel Wi-Fi signals coming into our house. Whenever the teenager next door texted on his deck, I felt a jolt. During World Series' commercials, when I figure people texted, I felt ripped. We installed EMF window shields, which helped some, but I still had constant pain. I told our neighbors about my problem and asked if they would move their Wi-Fi routers or get cabled access. Some said yes; others said no. Twice, I put up walls on our property to block Wi-Fi signals, but each time, the wall simply reflected cell phone coverage into our house. Installing Stetzer filters gave me significant relief. Within a few short years, I spent $30,000 trying reduce my exposure and stay in my house.

In August, 2010, PG&E sent notices around our neighborhood that they would install "smart" meters. I phoned repeatedly, but they refused to talk with me. I panicked. I did not know how to protect myself from a transmitting utility meter. For a significant loss, we sold our dream house.

Then came the question, Where do we go? *Since 2006, I've looked for respite from RF radiation all over the country and in Mexico. I have not found a place. I have resources, but I can't know where "smart" meters or cell towers will get installed or whether neighbors would work with me. I know of no place that legally prevents military, TV and radio satellites or wall-to-wall 4G.*

Wi-Fi and Health

Common symptoms from being around Wi-Fi include headaches, fatigue, nausea, rashes, and difficulty sleeping.

According to epidemiologist Samuel Milham, MD, MPH, "When industry apologists say that fields (like Wi-Fi) are too weak to cause biological effects, I point them to any number of electro-therapeutic devices, such as pulsed high-frequency field generators, that accelerate the healing of bone fractures. Anything that can stimulate cell division and growth is a potential carcinogen."[44]

In isolated human cells, Wi-Fi-like signals can activate the "cell suicide" response.[45]

According to environmental consultant Stan Hartman, having a Wi-Fi antenna in a router on your desk gives you about the same amount of radiation that you would get thirty meters or less from a typical cellular antenna.[46]

In 2006, the Simcoe County School District in Ontario, Canada installed Wi-Fi. Since that time, in at least fourteen of the district's schools have students who became ill with speeding heart rate, fatigue, and headaches. Two teenaged students had cardiac arrests and went on heart medication. "Now," Rodney Palmer, spokesman for the Simcoe Safe School Committee, reported to Canada's Parliamentary Standing Committee on Health in December, 2010, "every school in Simcoe

44 S. Milham, MD, MPH, *Dirty Electricity*, iUniverse.com, 2010.

45 S. Leea et al, "2.45 GHz radio frequency fields alter gene expression in cultured human cells," *FEBS Letters*, vol. 579 (2005): 4,829.

46 C. Reese and M. Havas, *Public Health SOS*, 2009.

County has its own defibrillator, as though teenage heart attacks are normal."[47]

ꕥ

Andrew Goldsworthy, PhD biologist, UK: *Like mobile phone signals, Wi-Fi signals can be expected to cause cell membranes to leak and calcium ions to flow through them in a relatively uncontrolled way. In the classroom, this may result in children's brains losing the ability to concentrate. Wi-Fi should therefore be considered an impediment to learning, rather than an aid. Wi-Fi may be particularly hazardous to pregnant teachers, since exposing the brain of a fetus or a very young child to EMR prevents normal brain development. Autism may result.*[48]

Effects on the nervous system are equally damaging since hyperactivity here can cause sensations such as pain, heat, cold and pins and needles. Hyperactivity in the cells of the inner ear can cause tinnitus (ringing in the ears). It can affect the sense of balance, causing dizziness and symptoms of motion sickness, including nausea. Students showing any of these symptoms should be treated with sympathy, and the Wi-Fi should be switched off.

Because of genetic and environmental variability, not everyone will suffer the same symptoms. Some may not suffer at all. For the sake of those who do suffer, Wi-Fi is not a good idea in schools—or anywhere else for that matter. Hard-wired cabled access is a healthier choice.

---

47 J. Nelson, "Jumping off the wireless bandwagon," *The Monitor,* Canadian Center for Policy Alternatives, 3-1-2011; also see www.safeschool.ca.

48 J. F. Krey, "Molecular mechanisms of autism: A possible role for Ca2+ signaling," *Current Opinion in Neurobiology,* vol. 17 , no. 1 (2007): 112–119.

Radio-Frequency Signals and Autism

In a 2013 paper in *Pathophysiology*, Harvard pediatric neurologist Dr. Martha Herbert and *BioInitiative Report* coeditor Cindy Sage write that "dramatic increases in reported Autism Spectrum Conditions (ASC)...are coincident in time with the deployment of wireless technologies." They outline evidence of plausible links between ASC and exposure to "low-intensity (non-thermal)" EMF/RFR levels. For example, "EMF/RFR exposure during pregnancy may send spurious signals to developing brain cells during pregnancy, altering brain development during critical periods, and may increase oxidative stress and immune reactivity that can increase risk for later developmental impairments, with further disruption later in development increasing risk, physiological dysregulation and severity of outcome."

Herbert and Sage clarify that while their paper "does not prove that EMF/RFR exposures cause autism...it does raise concerns that they could contribute by increasing risk, and by making challenging biological problems and symptoms worse in these vulnerable individuals." They urge schools, physicians and parents to take precautionary measures and provide children wired (not wireless) learning, living, and sleeping environments.

❈

Dr. Goldsworthy: *Some genetic forms of Autistic Spectrum Disorders (ASD) can be accounted for by known mutations in genetic coding for ion channels that result in an increased background concentration of calcium in neurons. This would be expected to lead to neuronal hyperactivity and the formation of sometimes inappropriate synapses, which in turn can lead to ASD.*[49]

49 T. Hawley and M. Gunner, "How early experiences affect brain development" (2000), http://tinyurl.com/5u23ae.

Before and just after birth, a child's brain is essentially a blank canvas. Then it goes through an intense period of becoming aware of new sensory input—e.g., recognizing its mother's face, her expressions, and eventually other people and their relationship to him or her.[50] *During this process, the neurons in the brain make countless new connections, and the brain stores what the child learns. After a few months, connections that are rarely used are pruned. The patterns that remain could become hard-wired into the child's psyche.*

If the child is exposed to radio frequencies during this period, the production of too many and often spurious signals will generate frequent random connections. These will not be pruned, even though they may not make sense. Because the pruning process in children exposed to RFs may be more random, these children—who may have more brain cells than the rest of us and may actually be savants—may lack the mindset for normal patterns of social interaction. This may then contribute to the various autistic spectrum disorders.

How Is Exposure to Radiation from Microwave Ovens Different from Radiation Emitted by Telecommunications?

Microwave ovens operate at 2.4 GHz. But they're used only for short periods and are shielded to prevent leakage—although they always leak slightly through their windows. (To test leakage on your microwave oven, unplug it, put a mobile phone inside and close the door. If the phone can receive a call, your oven probably leaks.)

Typically, Wi-Fi transmits, at 2.4 GHz. Because of widespread deployment of wireless devices, telecom antennas and "smart" meters, people are now constantly exposed to RFs

50 P. R. Huttenlocher and A. S. Dabholkar, "Regional differences in synaptogenesis in human cerebral cortex," *Journal of Comparative Neurology,* vol. 387, no. 2 (1997): 167–178.

between 800 MHz and 2.4 GHz.[51] These frequencies are new for humans and wildlife: they are not found in nature. It's also worth noting that cellular antennas require power supplies that may affect the power quality of nearby electrical systems.

How Does Living Near a Cellular Antenna (a Base Station) Affect Health?

Studies find that people living near a base station experience fatigue, headache, sleep disruption, irritability, depression, decreased libido, memory loss, dizziness, nausea, increased risk of cancer, tremors, loss of appetite, rashes, visual disruptions and overall discomfort.[52]

People who live within 350 meters of a cellular antenna for more than a decade experience a four-fold increase in cancer rates. Among women, the increase is tenfold.[53,]

People who live within 200 to 500 feet of an antenna report genetic, growth and reproductive effects; increases in the permeability of the blood–brain barrier; behavioral, molecular, cellular, and metabolic effects; and an increased risk of cancer.[54]

---

51 R. Santini et al, "Survey study of people living in the vicinity of cellular phone base stations," *Electromagnetic Biology and Medicine* vol. 22, no. 1 (2003): 41–49.

52 B. Levitt and H. Lai, "Biological effects from exposure to electromagnetic radiation emitted by cell tower base stations and other antenna arrays," *Environmental Reviews*, vol. 18 (2010): 369–395. H. P. Hutter et al, "Mobile phone base stations: Effects on health and wellbeing," *Pathophysiology*, vol. 16 nos. 2–3 (2009): 123–135.

53 R. Wolf and D. Wolf, "Increased incidence of cancer near a cellphone transmitted station," *International Journal of Cancer Prevention*, vol. 1, no. 2 (2004). Review by M. Kundi, "Evidence for childhood cancers (leukemia), brain tumor epidemiology, III: Epidemiological studies of RF and brain tumors," C. Selvin et al, "The BioInitiative Report: A Rationale for a Biologically-based Public Exposure Standard for Electromagnetic Fields" (http://www.bioinitiative.org/).

54 B. Levitt, ibid.

In Brazil, from 1996 to 2006, researchers tracked people who lived within 500 meters of a base station. They found 34.76 deaths by neoplasia (some kind of tumor) per 10,000 inhabitants. Outside of this area, a *decrease* in the number of deaths by neoplasia occurred: the greatest incidence was 5.83 deaths per 1,000 people.[55]

In Israel, living near a cellular antenna for one year led to a dramatic increase of cancer. The increase correlates with previous data on significant increase in leukemia among people who live near broadcasting towers in Honolulu[56] and Hawaii.[57]

Egyptian researchers found that long-term (six years) exposure to cellular antennas and mobile phones negatively impacts human hormone profiles: cortisol, serum progesterone (in females), and thyroid hormones are all affected.[58]

After a cellular antenna was installed in Rimbach, a small town in Bavaria, Germany, sixty residents had their urine tested regularly over eighteen months, beginning in Spring, 2004. Participants' stress hormones (adrenaline and noradrenaline) increased significantly; their dopamine and phenylethylamine levels decreased substantially. While participants maintained their usual lifestyle, they experienced increases in sleep problems,

---

55 A. C. Dode et al, "Mortality by neoplasia and cellular telephone base stations in the Belo Horizonte municipality, Minas Gerais state, Brazil," *Science of the Total Environment*, vol. 409, no. 19 (2011), 3,649–3,665

56 J. R. Goldsmith, "Epidemiologic evidence of radio frequency radiation (microwave) effects on health in military, broadcasting, and occupational studies," *International Journal of Occupational and Environmental Health*, vol. 1, no. 1 (1995): 47–57.

57 G. Maskarinee et al, "Investigation of increased incidence in childhood leukemia near radio towers in Hawaii; preliminary observations," *Journal of Environmental Pathology, Toxicology and Oncology*, vol. 13, no. 1 (1994): 33–7.

58 E. F. Eskander et al, "How does long term exposure to base stations and mobile phones affect human hormone profiles?" *Clinical Biochemistry*, vol. 45, nos. 1–2 (2012): 157–161.

headaches, dizziness, concentration problems, and allergies. Because chronic disruption of hormones damages health in the long run, researchers expect "major health problems" from long-term exposure to radiation from cellular antennas.[59]

For an excellent film about living near an antenna, see "Resonance: Beings of Frequency" by James Russell, available for free at vimeo.com. To learn how many antennas are in your neighborhood, go to www.antennasearch.com and type in the address of your home, school, or workplace. Or, locate any type of transmitter at the FCC Dashboard: http://reboot.fee.gov/reform/systems/spectrum-dashboard.fcc.

"Smart" Meters and Health

In June 2012, in the Quebec-based magazine, *La maison du 21e siecle*, fifty-four scientists and health professionals from around the world released "Smart Meters: Correcting the Gross Misinformation." This statement explains that "if a smart meter is located on a wall with a bedroom or kitchen, the RF exposure can be the same as if you are within 200 to 600 feet of a cell tower with multiple carriers. With both cell towers and "smart" meters, the entire body is immersed by microwaves that go out in all directions, which increases the risk of overexposure to many sensitive organs, such as the eyes and testicles. With a cell phone, people are exposed to microwaves primarily in the head and neck (unless using speaker mode), and only when they use their device." These fifty-four scientists and medical experts urgently recommend a return to analog mechanical meters.

According to environmental consultants Sage Associates, "smart" meters violate the FCC public safety standards and endanger people with medical implants as well as developing

59 K. Buchner and H. Eger, , "Changes of clinically important neurotransmitters under the influence of modulated RF fields: A long-term study under real-life conditions," *Umwelt-Medizin-Gesellschaft*, vol. 24, no. 1 (2011): 44–57.

fetuses and children whose central nervous systems continue to develop into their late teens.[60]

For a video of a man whose pacemaker shut off after "smart" meters were installed around his neighborhood, go to youtube .com/watch?v=BRDhogkdxW4.

In Austin, Texas, Dr. Laura Pressley and her husband noticed that their legs twitched every 25 seconds at bedtime. A meter determined that the wireless utility meter near their bedroom also pulsed every 25 seconds.[61]

To refuse installation of a radiation-emitting surveillance device on your property or residence, see Jerry Day's letter in the appendix.

⌘

Judy Neal, 52, Northeast: *I had good health, a cell phone and Wi-Fi until September 2009. I work at home, but starting that month, I could not focus enough to work. I could not remember words or where I'd put things. Every night, I woke up several times, agitated. I was always on high alert. Privately, I wondered if I had Alzheimer's.*

In February 2010, during a winter storm, our electricity kept going off and on. I got a high-pitched, painful ring in my right ear. I started having heart palpitations and nightmares, and my other symptoms got stronger. I wondered if something was wrong with our electricity. My electrician wondered if my electric company had installed "one of those new meters" on our home. They had—in June 2009.

After several phone calls and a letter from my doctor, my electric company removed the transmitting "smart" meter.

60 Sage Associates, "Thirteen Flaws of Smart Meter Technology," 2011; www.sagereports.com.

61 See an interview with Dr. Pressley, "Is Your Smart Meter Causing Brain Damage?" at youtube.com/watch?v=dhF6C_pB22g&feature =em-uploadermail.

Within days, the pulsing and loud buzzing quieted, and my thinking got clear again. But now, if I am near a cell phone or Wi-Fi or if I drive by a cell tower, I get sharp pain in my head and pressure in my ears.

I consider the "smart" meter my tipping point. Unfortunately, my neighborhood is still flooded with them. Each one transmits pulses of microwave radiation 24/7. When I requested studies about the meters' effects on human health, my electric company told me I would need a subpoena.

In the fall of 2012, I compiled a list of friends and acquaintances in my town (population 8,000) who've gotten sick or died since transmitting meters were installed here:

- *Three men (48, 55, and 60) and one woman (70) died of a massive heart attack in 2009; previously, none of them was known to have a heart condition.*
- *Two women, who had each been in remission from breast cancer, had recurrences. One has died. The other is currently in treatment.*
- *Two women in their fifties committed suicide.*
- *One woman in her forties suffered a stroke.*
- *Several people now have high blood pressure and tinnitus, problems they did not have before.*

When I reported this at a city council meeting, members of a Boy Scout troop, attending for another matter, spoke up and said that they have headaches and cannot sleep. Then, a friend told me that she knows seven people newly diagnosed with cancer. In 2013, two more men in their 40s had heart attacks; one died.

We need independently funded studies about the health effects of these meters, including when they're installed on homes that have Wi-Fi, DECT cordless phones, fluorescent lights and/or digital appliances. States that have not yet installed them need to wait until such tests have been conducted, because too many people are getting sick.

⌘

Nannette Proctor, 39, Northwest: *After our town got "smart" meters, my husband went on anti-anxiety medication for the first time. Two years later, our twelve-year-old told me that she did not do well on tests because she could not remember what she had studied the night before.* That *sobered me. I got the "smart" meter removed from our house.*[62]

Other Health Effects of Electrification and Exposure to Wireless Devices

Diabetes

Until the 1950s, childhood type 1 diabetes was rare. Soon after the middle of the century, epidemiologists noted a rapid increase in the disease. Within a genetically stable population, a rapid change suggests that children were reared differently, or that something in their environment has changed.[63] Could electrification have contributed to the increase in childhood diabetes?

In a 2013 paper, epidemiologist Samuel Milham, MD, wrote, "The epidemics of obesity and diabetes, most apparent in recent years, had their origins with Thomas Edison's development of distributed electricity in New York City in 1882. His original direct current (DC) generators suffered serious brush arcing, which is a major source of high-frequency voltage transients (dirty electricity). From the onset of the electrical grid, electrified populations have been exposed to dirty electricity. Diesel generator sets are a major source of dirty electricity today and

62 For a catalog of symptoms reported by ratepayers after "smart" meter installation, go to EmfSafetyNetwork.org.

63 E. A. Gale, "The rise of childhood type 1 diabetes in the 20th century," *Diabetes*, vol. 51, no. 12 (2002): 3,353–3,361.

are used almost universally to electrify small islands and places unreachable by the conventional electric grid. This accounts for the fact that diabetes prevalence, fasting plasma glucose and obesity are highest on small islands and other places electrified by generator sets and lowest in places with low levels of electrification, like sub-Saharan Africa and east and Southeast Asia."[64]

Anton Mark, 37, Midwest: *Doctors don't really know why the immune system attacks the pancreas and causes Type I diabetes. I was diagnosed with it at eleven. I've wondered if exposure to high frequency fields could cause the disease, at least in part.*

When the house I grew up in was built, no one expected to use more electricity than it took to operate a few lightbulbs. Starting in the late seventies, my parents gradually rewired the house's inside. But the wires coming from the utility service—installed in the 1940s—were not replaced. Eventually, the insulation on these wires hung in shreds, and a pine tree grew into them. Each time a pine needle touched a wire, the house got an arcing event. Looking back, the tree likely started hitting the electrical wires in the year or two before I was diagnosed with diabetes, and my mother was diagnosed with rheumatoid arthritis.

My slender, active sister was recently diagnosed with Type I diabetes at 28. In the years before her diagnosis, she had a wireless router on the wall beside her bed and became very attached to her cell phone. At the time of her diagnosis, her home had two "smart" meters.

Is her diabetes a coincidence? Perhaps. But on an extended backwoods hike that she took after her diagnosis, she needed almost no insulin.

---

64 S. Milham, "Evidence that dirty electricity is causing the worldwide epidemic of obesity and diabetes," *Electromagnetic Biology and Medicine*, vol. 33, no. 1 (2014); 75–78.

I switched from insulin shots to a pump to improve my blood-sugar control at twenty-three. As a farmer, I'm not often around wireless devices. No coworkers' cell phones; no close neighbors with Wi-Fi. A few years ago, I visited friends who turned off their wireless router during my stay. Then, a couple of hours before I left, they turned it back on. My blood sugar jumped to 260. Normally, I try to keep it between 80 and 120.

Visiting my sister's home, my blood sugar soared to 360 and stayed there in spite of repeated doses of insulin.

Another time, I harvested corn for a neighbor. For three hours, he and his cell phone rode with me in the cab of a combine. I started to feel unwell and agitated, so I tested my blood sugar. It was close to 300, and would not come down, even as I took appropriate doses of insulin. Once my neighbor and his cell phone left the combine and my insulin began to work, my blood sugar dropped like a rock to 30—dangerously low. I had to drink several cans of root beer to bring it back to safe levels.

In my experience, radio-frequency signals from wireless devices impair the action of insulin, stress the pancreas, and impair and hyperactivate the immune system. Certainly, I do not like subjecting myself to dangerous extremes, which wireless devices appear to cause. To safeguard my health, limiting my exposure to cell phones and Wi-Fi now means limiting my participation in society.

I'm a slender, physically active man. Does my experience explain why diabetes has become a national epidemic?

Along with Dr. Milham's observations, a 2009 email to the EMR Policy Institute responds to Anton's question. Richard Whitehead, a concerned citizen, compared the percentage of people in seven industrialized countries who had insulin-dependent diabetes from 1993 to 1994[65] with the percentage of people who had cell phones in 1995.[66] Whitehead found:

Country	Diabetes rate	Cell phone use
Finland	36%	24.7%
Denmark	22%	21.9%
Norway	21%	24.6%
Great Britain	13%	10.2%
The United States	9%	14.4%
France	8%	2.9%
Germany	7%	5.7%

"Generally, but not exactly," Mr. Whitehead observed, "the insulin-dependent diabetes rate coincides with the cell phone penetration rate. Of course, this doesn't prove a relationship, but when considered along with the 1994 study by Navakatikian showing a serious drop in insulin caused by radio frequency non-ionizing radiation, it certainly looks suspicious. It is also interesting," he continues, "that diabetes has increased steadily in recent years, right along with the increase in radiation-producing technology. Diabetes is often thought to be caused by obesity, but the obesity rate in the above countries does not coincide with the diabetes rate at all. According to the International Obesity Task Force,[67] England, Germany, and Finland's obesity rates are 40 to 45%. The U.S. is about 50%. France, Sweden, and Norway are around 20 to 25%.

65 Data from "Prevalence and incidence of insulin-dependent diabetes" by R. E. LaPorte et al, http://diabetes.niddk.nih.gov/dm/pubs/america/pdf/chapter3.pdf.

66 Statistics are from IDATE World Atlas of Mobiles/Washingtonpost.com 1995 data.

67 See www.obesity.chair.ulaval.ca/ITOF.htm.

Whitehead also noted an article that appeared in the November 16, 2000, *Christian Science Monitor,* "Two Border Cities Seek End to Communications Chaos." The article described an enormous proliferation of mobile phone usage and, thereby, cellular antennas, in Laredo, Texas. Meanwhile, the Laredo Health Department found an unusually high diabetes rate among their citizens. At the February 7, 2000, Laredo City Council meeting, Councilman Joe. A. Guerro stated that "Webb County has the highest death rate due to diabetes." Webb County's death rate from diabetes was 55.5 out of 100,000, while the average rate for counties on Texas' western border (including Webb) was 43.6.[68]

⌘

Emma Gunn, 31, Pennsylvania: *At twelve, I was diagnosed with type 1 diabetes, even though I ate very little sugar as a child. We had organic, homemade meals, fresh fruit and vegetables for snacks. I think I got the disease because my mother had dental mercury removed while she was pregnant with me, and then I had several vaccines in my early childhood.*

A few years ago, I got an insulin pump to help steady my blood sugar levels. Still, I find myself in precarious situations several times each month. If my blood sugar level gets too low, I can lose consciousness. I need juice or glucagon. I may need to call for help.

Before I had a cell phone, having type 1 diabetes meant that I needed another person and/or a landline near me at all times. I still have a landline, but the cell phone lets me be independent and mobile.

Recently, I've learned about the hazards of RFs and magnetic fields. I see that there are no easy answers—for me or for anyone. I have to admit that even with all I've learned—and

68 See www.ci.laredo.tx.us/city-council/council-activities/council-minutes/2000Min/M2000-R-04.html.

the fact that I get a headache if I use my cell phone for more than a minute, I don't feel able to let go of it.

Allergies, Rashes, Asthma, and Cellular Inflammation

In May 2013, the Centers for Disease Control and Prevention reported that one in eight children now has eczema and other skin allergies, an increase of 69% from a survey conducted in the late 1990s. About one in twenty children now has food allergies, a 50% increase from the earlier survey. Dr. Lara Akinbami, the report's senior author, says that researchers don't know the cause of these dramatic increases.[69]

Dr. Hajime Kimata, who has published research in the *International Archives of Allergy and Immunology*, says that mobile phones raise the levels of certain chemicals in the blood. These chemicals "provoke allergic reactions such as eczema, hay fever and asthma. Mobile phone radiation can 'excite' antigens—substances that cause allergies—in the bloodstream of people who already suffer from allergies."[70]

To hear cardiologist Stephen Sinatra, MD discuss why radiation from wireless devices is the number one cause of cell inflammation, how human-made EMFs cause cell death and can lead to brain cancer, heart disease, chronic fatigue, fibromyalgia, and more, go to www.heartmdinstitute.com/v1/wireless-safety/cordless-phone-use-can-affect-heart.

Neurological Diseases, Including Dementia

While mortality rates in twenty Western countries have decreased in the last few decades, death by neurological diseases

69 J. Silverberg et al, "Prevalence of allergic disease in foreign-born American children," *JAMA Pediatrics*, vol. 167, no. 6 (2013) 554–560. M. Stobbe, "Study: Food, skin allergies increasing among children," Associated Press, May 2, 2013.

70 See www.healthandgoodness.com/article/cell-phone-radiation-and-allergies.html.

such as Parkinson's, motor neuron disease, hereditary neuromuscular conditions, prion disorders, degenerative diseases and Alzheimer's has increased. Some countries report increasing rates of dementia, as well as early onset dementia and increasingly younger patients with motor neuron disease. In looking for potential environmental explanations, several British scientists suggested that "increased home technology involving increased background electromagnetic fields" from mobile phones, microwave ovens, computers, etc. might be involved.[71]

Meanwhile, in South Korea (perhaps the world's most digitally connected country, where more than 67% of the population has a smartphone and more than 64% of teenagers have one), doctors report a surge in "digital dementia" among young people: they have become so dependent on electronic devices that they can't remember details like their own phone numbers. Doctors are witnessing deterioration in young peoples' cognitive abilities that is similar to people who have suffered a head injury or a psychiatric illness. Dr. Byun Gi-won, a physician at Seoul's Balance Brain Center, told the *JoongAng Daily* that heavy users of smartphones and game devices are likely to develop the left and right sides of their brains disproportionately, leaving the right side "untapped or undeveloped."[72]

Addiction to Mobile Devices

Addiction is compulsive behavior beyond an individual's control. When does use of a substance such as alcohol or a painkiller—*or* a behavior like using a cell phone—become an unhealthy addiction? Typically, psychologists consider the frequency of use, the amount of money spent on it, and the

71 C. Pritchard et al, "Changing patterns of neurological mortality in the 10 major developed countries 1979–2010," *Royal Society for Public Health*, vol. 127, no. 4 (2013): 357–368.

72 See www.telegraph.co.uk/news/worldnews/asia/southkorea/10138403/Surge-in-digital-dementia.html/.

degree to which the use interferes with family, social, and work relationships.

Addictive behavior is based in neurophysiology: the drug or behavior acts on the brain's neurotransmitters by creating pleasurable sensations and a "reward" system that keeps the user using more. The substance or behavior signals the brain that it (i.e., getting a text) is beneficial, which moves the user to increase message-checking.[73] This mechanism, sometimes called the dopamine effect, is not accessible to the conscious mind.

Microwaves (frequencies required for mobile devices to operate) increase activity of brain endorphins or endogenous opioids, which are the biological base of addiction to opium, alcohol, and morphine.[74]

Exposure to radio-frequency fields activates benzodiazepine receptors (which relate to anxiety and stress responses) in a rat's brain.[75] The RFs probably reinforce the euphoric qualities of opiates. The brain's neurotransmitters are sensitive to weak, modulated microwaves—such as those found in cell phone radiation.[76] Whole body exposure (like that experienced around

---

73 J. Tirapu et al, 2004.

74 M. Paz de la Puent and A. Balmori, "Addiction to cell phones: Are there neurophysiologic mechanisms involved?" *Proyecto*, vol. 61 (Mar. 2007): 8–12: in English at emfacts.com.

75 C. Braestrup et al, "Benzodiazepine receptors in the brain as affected by different experimental stresses: The changes are small and not unidirectional," *Psychopharmacology* (Berlin), vol. 65 no. 3 (1979): 273–277; H. Lai et al, "Single vs. repeated microwave exposure: Effects on benzodiazepine receptors in the brain of the rat," *Bioelectromagnetics* vol. 13, no. 1, (1992): 57–66; B. M. Walker and A. Ettenberg, "Benzodiazepine modulation of opiate reward," *Experimental and Clinical Psychopharmacology*, vol. 9 no. 2 (2001): 191–197, .

76 W. R. Adey, "Electromagnetic fields, the modulation of brain tissue functions: A possible paradigm shift in biology," in G. Adelman and B. Smith (eds.), *International Encyclopedia of Neuroscience*, 2003.

"smart" meters, Wi-Fi, and/or a security system) can also activate endogenous opioids in the brain.[77]

How do these scientific discoveries relate to real lives? In 2006, 90% of 106 students surveyed at the University of Staffordshire in Stoke-on-Trent in UK admitted that they took their phones everywhere. Nearly 40% said that they could not cope without their cell phone. Thirty-five percent said that they used mobile devices to escape their problems. Seven percent blamed their phone for the loss of a significant relationship or job.[78] Dr. David Sheffield, who administered the survey, likened such cell phone use to a gambling addiction. He also found that when the students used their cell phones less, their blood pressure lowered.[79]

In 2008, at the University of Northampton in the UK, Nada Kakabadse, a professor at the Northampton Business School, found that one third of the workers she surveyed who used a mobile phone for work showed signs of addiction similar to alcoholics. At first, using a mobile phone made workers very productive, but then they became very anxious if their gadget was not nearby.[80]

What are other characteristics of addiction to portable technology?

- a compulsion to reply to each new message, which leads to tiring and slowing down the brain.

77 H. Lai et al, " Intraseptal microinjection of beta-funaltrexamine blocked a microwave-induced decrease of hippocampal cholinergic activity in the rat," *Pharmacology Biochemistry and Behavior* vol. 53, no. 3 (1994): 613–616; M.A. Rojavin and M. C. Ziskin, "Electromagnetic millimeter waves increase the duration of anesthesia caused by ketamine and chloral hydrate in mice," *International Journal of Radiation Biology*, vol. 72, no. 4, (1997): 475–480.

78 See www.msnbc.msn.com/id/14832639/.

79 M. Paz de la Puente and A. Balmori, "Addition to cell phones," ibid.

80 Forbes.com.staff04.03.08.

- spending more time with a mobile device than with family.
- the time between work and play becomes blurred so that the work-week never ends.
- the overwork leads to more stress and tiredness, less intimacy, more conflict with partners and premature career burnout.
- decision-making processes and judgments are impaired.[81]
- *nomophobia*, fear of being without a phone, increases.[82]
- people are always partly somewhere else.

In Spain, in 2008, two children, ages twelve and thirteen, were admitted to a clinic for addiction because they had lied to relatives in order to get money for phones. They'd become irritable, antisocial, and their schoolwork had deteriorated. Dr. Jose Martinez-Raga, an addictions expert, warned that these cases could be "the tip of the iceberg."[83]

Even toddlers now show signs of addiction to mobile devices. In 2013, a four-year-old who used an iPad up to four hours each day became "distressed and inconsolable" whenever her parents took the device away from her. The parents enrolled her in digital detox. According to Dr. Richard Graham, founder of London's Capio Nightingale Clinic, when their devices are taken away, young technology addicts experience the same withdrawal symptoms as alcoholics or heroin addicts.[84]

In a 2013 survey of more than one thousand parents conducted by www.babies.co.uk, more than half allowed their babies to play with mobile phones and tablets. One in seven

81 See www.news.bbc.co.uk/1/hi/programmes/click_online/6411495.stm.

82 "Rise in Nomophobia: Fear of Being without a Phone," www.telegraph.co.uk/news, 2.16.12.

83 See www.news.bbc.co.uk/go/pr/fr/-2/hi/europe/7452463.stm.

84 See www.telegraph.co.uk/technology/10008707/Toddlers-becoming-so-addicted-to-iPads-they-require-therapy.html.

parents admitted that they let their babies use the devices for four or more hours per day.[85]

ꕤ

Cindy Sage, M.A., Coeditor of the *BioInitiative Reports*, environmental consultant: *If the use of cell phones is physiologically addictive, then these devices need to be classified as drug delivery systems and regulated as such. Certainly children should not use them at all until this mechanism is more fully understood.*

Medical Implants

A brochure from pacemaker manufacturer Biotronik states that "pacemakers are protected against the impact of electric devices and their radiation to the greatest extent possible. However, if you should experience symptoms, such as increased heartbeat, irregular pulse or dizziness in the vicinity of electric devices, please move away from the device immediately and/or turn off the external device." The brochure also says, "You can use (a cellular) phone without hesitation." And, it states, "If you want to use a cellular phone, you should talk to your physician. To prevent possible interference, you should always hold the cell phone at the side opposite from the implanted pacemaker. *Even when not in use* (emphasis added) you should not keep it close to the pacemaker."

Testing and regulation of the effects of interference on medical implants are long overdue. After he had a DBS implanted for Parkinson's, a man drove his hybrid car. Each time the car's charging system came on at a stoplight, his DBS shut off.

ꕤ

85 Ibid.

Gary Olhoeft, PhD, geophysicist and electrical engineer: *The Medtronic manual for my deep brain stimulator (implanted to ease effects of Parkinson's) lists more than sixteen pages of potential electromagnetic interferences. I have experienced interference with the operation and programming of my medical implant in elevators, on large commercial aircraft, at malls, libraries, government buildings and other places with security systems. Because interferences are almost everywhere, I built a monitor to carry around and warn me of potential hazards to avoid, including security and inventory control systems, Wi-Fi, "smart" meters, cell and radio/TV towers, wireless phones and wireless devices, buildings with faulty wiring, light dimmers, certain appliances, and many more.*

If I walk through a security system—like the ones commonly found in retail stores, airports, government buildings or in the library at the university where I teach—my DBS sometimes shuts off. I have four seconds to reset it or I shake so badly that I am unable to reset it without help.

The National Institute of Health estimates that twenty-five million Americans now have implanted medical devices. Besides brain stimulators, the functioning of cardiac pacemakers, insulin pumps, cochlear implants and bone stimulators can also be disturbed by RF signals. A disabled person's getting x-rayed while sitting in a metal wheelchair can be especially dangerous.

A friend with an insulin pump has to shut it off when he flies, because his pump interferes with the plane's avionics, and they interfere with his pump. This limits how far he can travel. A former student told me that if she's around several people using cell phones, her insulin pump malfunctions.

After another friend with a brain stimulator and *a pacemaker had a cochlear implant installed, the signals from his implants interfered with each other. Each device functioned inappropriately, and he experienced tremendous discomfort. The surgeons who installed the devices suggested that his home's electrical system was the source of his trouble. They did not believe that implants could interfere with each other. They can. Unfortunately, medical implants are not regulated for such interference; and my friend—who is an MD—had to prove to his physicians that they were causing him trouble.*

Recently, at a meeting of people with brain stimulators for Parkinson's, I asked if any of their implants shut off when they walk through security doors at malls and other places. Fifty people were in the room. Everyone raised a hand.

But no agency studies the effects of radio-frequency signals on medical implants. Even doctors who implant devices are likely unaware of the problems—though implant manufacturers typically alert patients to pages of dangers in their manuals.

Medical Equipment

Medical equipment—including fetal monitors used in hospitals and cardiac pacemakers as well as sensitive, personal medical information—has become vulnerable to hackers. Increasingly, computer viruses and "malware" infect computers that view X-rays and CT scans; they can cause equipment to slow down or shut off. In 2010 and 2011, several hospitals temporarily closed their cardiac catheterization labs (which widen blocked arteries), because of infected devices.[86]

According to John Halamka, chief information officer of Boston's Beth Israel Deaconess Medical Center, on a typical day, the hospital runs about 15,000 devices on its computer network. About 500 of these devices use older operating systems that are

86 See www.washingtonpost.com/national/health-science/facing-cybersecurity-threats-fda-tightens-medical-device-standards-2013/06/12/b79ccofe-d3jo-11e2-b051-3ea310e7bb5a_story.html.

especially susceptible to malware infections beyond the hospital's direct control.[87]

In August 2012, the U.S. Government Accountability Office reported that defibrillators and insulin pumps are vulnerable to hacks.

To access hospital computers that hold patient records, physicians need to enter their password at various computers, sometimes hourly. When a nurse keeps a doctor "logged in" and when computers are left unattended, sensitive medical information becomes vulnerable.[88]

Medical equipment may also affect health.

❈

Katharine J. Lee, 66, New Mexico: *At 38, I was diagnosed with multiple sclerosis (MS). Call it an electrical problem: there's miscommunication between my brain and the rest of my body. At 57, I got a power wheelchair. It frees me to use my stamina for things other than rock-bottom essentials. It also means that I sit on two batteries every day and charge them several nights each week. I sense that the digital electronics, the batteries and their recharging are potentially harmful to me. But even with the risks involved, the power chair gives me so many benefits that I can't imagine living without it.*

Is there a way to shield myself from the batteries? Would filters make my electrical system safer while the batteries charge? Where can I go for information about this?

❈

Emma Gunn, 31, Type 1 diabetic, Pennsylvania: *In the spring of 2013, I got a stomach virus. After nearly twenty-four hours of vomiting, I went to the hospital. In the ICU, I was wired to*

---

87 Ibid.

88 Ibid.

several monitors and a digitalized IV drip that gave me anti-nausea medication and another drug (that I am usually on) to raise my blood pressure. For four days, vomiting and dry heaves continued. When my blood pressure went up to 166/115, the drug that raises blood pressure was stopped. I was given another drug that lowers it. I could barely talk.

On Day 4, the virus began to subside. The time between vomiting got longer. I moved out of the ICU into a room that did not have a wired heart monitor—only a wireless one. This room also had a view of a cell tower about a quarter of a mile away. My health continued to improve, but I felt that the wireless monitor kept me from fully regaining my strength.

My mother told the doctor that Dr. Magda Havas, a medical researcher, found that blood-sugar control[89] *and blood pressure*[90] *are affected by the radio-frequency signals that wireless devices use to operate. She asked if he could remove the wireless heart monitor.*

Hospital policy states that when blood-pressure meds are delivered intravenously, the patient must wear a heart monitor. This good doctor realized that if I took the medication orally, then he could remove the wireless monitor.

My blood pressure normalized as soon as the monitor came off. I left the hospital the next day. My doctor wondered whether other patients are affected by wireless and digitalized equipment.

Indeed, I wonder how exposure to such equipment affected me. I wonder how medical workers are affected since they're

---

89 M. Havas, "Dirty electricity elevates blood sugar among electrically sensitive diabetics and may explain brittle diabetes," *Electromagnetic Biology and Medicine*, vol. 27, no. 2 (2008): 135–146.

90 M. Havas et al, "Provocation study using heart rate variability shows microwave radiation from 2.4 GHz cordless phones affects autonomic nervous system," *European Journal of Oncology*, vol. 5, (2010): 273–300.

exposed to wireless transmitting medical equipment throughout the work week—along with cell towers, Wi-Fi, fluorescent lights and wireless keyboards. I wonder what my options are if I get dangerously sick again.

While the FDA has the authority to regulate digitalized and wireless medical devices, Congress does not provide the funding to do so.

In the U.S., Canada, and Sweden, some hospitals have designated low-EMF zones.

Fertility

Fertility is the ability to reproduce. The quality of fertility matters to the health of every family—and to every community's survival. Every family and community that welcomes a baby wants him or her healthy—and for parents to keep healthy at least until their children reach adulthood. To begin, then, women need healthy menstrual cycles. Men need erectile function and healthy sperm. Women need healthy pregnancies.

In 1997, I began teaching natural family planning (NFP), a method of birth control also used as an aid for those who want to conceive. Based on charting a woman's waking temperature and cervical fluid, the method provides women an accurate way of knowing when they are fertile and infertile. By 2004, when my book, *The Garden of Fertility*, was published, one third of my NFP students were not ovulating. This correlated with national statistics about the percentage of women of childbearing age who had polycystic ovarian syndrome, a condition in which the woman ovulates infrequently or not at all. In *The Garden*, I also reported the detrimental effects of pharmaceutical family planning, of sleeping exposed to light (i.e., from a TV or a street lamp)—as well as the benefits of sleeping in darkness and a nutrient-dense diet.

In 2007, the biologist Sandra Steingraber wrote "The Falling Age of Puberty in U.S. Girls." She reported that girls have begun to menstruate at younger and younger ages (and the early onset of menses increases a woman's risk of breast cancer). Among other factors, Steingraber reported that early puberty is caused by girls' watching television.

In the few years since these publications, use of electronics, wireless devices and wireless services has increased exponentially. So have my questions: What happens to a girl's reproductive health if she gets exposed to first- or second-hand cell phone radiation before she menstruates? How are menstrual cycles and offsprings' health affected if a teenaged girl sleeps exposed to Wi-Fi? If she sleeps with a mobile device under her pillow or keeps a phone in her bra? What are the effects of using a cell phone or sleeping near a Wi-Fi router while taking the Pill (or other pharmaceutical birth control)? What are the long-term health effects when people are exposed to cell phones, Wi-Fi, broadband over power lines, "smart" meters, and other radiation-emitting devices from conception onward? How is long-term reproductive health affected when children attend school with fluorescent lights, wireless tablets, and Wi-Fi routers?

I do not know of studies that answer these questions. In India, the Council of Medical Research has begun studying how use of a cell phone or proximity to a cell tower impacts a woman's menstrual cycle and a man's sperm count, as well as their sleep patterns and general behavior.

Meanwhile, here's what studies that we do have report: Numerous studies show that sperm quality and motility are adversely affected when men wear a cell phone, PDA, or pager on their belt or in a pocket.[91] Yet other studies conclude that

91 A. Agarwal et. al, "Effect of cell phone usage on semen analysis in men attending infertility clinic: an observational study," *Fertility and Sterility,* vol. 92, no. 1, (2008): 124–128; and "Effects of radio frequency electromagnetic waves (RF-EMW) from cellular phones on

using a cell phone or storing one near the testes affects sperm counts, motility, viability, and structure.[92]

The 2012 Proceeding of the World Meeting on Sexual Medicine reports that men with erectile dysfunction are 2.6 times more likely to keep their cell phones in their front pants pocket. (Researchers did not consider different types of phones, nor the amount of time that the man had kept his phone in his pocket.)

After five generations of exposure to RF radiation from cell towers (less than one microwatt per centimeter squared), mice become irreversibly infertile.[93]

An increase in deep vein thrombosis as the leading cause of death in pregnancy now has researchers wondering about its connection with the growing use of mobile phones during pregnancy.[94]

A new study associates mothers using mobile phones and computers during pregnancy with pre-term births.[95]

---

human ejaculated semen: an in vitro pilot study," *Fertility and Sterility,* vol. 92, no. 4 (2009): 318–325; A. Wdowiak et al, "Evaluation of the effect of using mobile phones on male fertility," *Annals of Agricultural and Environmental Medicine,* vol. 14, no. 1 (2007): 69–172; G. N. De Iuliis et al, "Mobile phone radiation induces reactive oxygen species production and DNA damage in human spermatozoa in vitro," *PLoS One*, vol. 4, no. 7 (2009): e6446; I. Fejes et al, 2005, "Is there a relationship between cell phone use and sperm quality?" *Archives of Andrology,* vol. 51, no. 5 (2005): 385–393.

92 R. J. Aitken et al, "Seeds of concern," *Nature*, vol. 432 (2004): 48–52; O. Erogul et al, "Effects of electromagnetic radiation from a cellular phone on human sperm motility: an in vitro study," *Archives of Medical Research*, vol. 37, no. 7 (2006): 840–843.

93 I. N. Magras and T. D. Xenos, "RF radiation-induced changes in the prenatal development of mice," *Bioelectromagnetics,* vol. 18, no. 6 (1997): 455–461.

94 D. I. Davis et al, "Swedish review strengthens grounds for concluding that radiation from cellular and cordless phones is a probable human carcinogen," *Pathophysiology* vol. 20, no. 2 (2013): 123–129.

95 N. Col-Araz, "Evaluation of factors affecting birth weight and preterm birth in southern Turkey," *Journal of Pakistan Medical*

Five Danish Ninth-Graders Experiment

In early 2013, five ninth-graders from the Hjallerup School in Denmark noticed that they often had difficulty concentrating in school if they slept the night before with a mobile phone near their head. The young women's question about how radiation emitted by cell phones affects people led to an experiment that tested the effect of two routers (which the students determined emitted about the same amount of radiation as a cell phone) on garden cress. The students put six trays of cress seeds in a room with two routers, and six trays in a room without routers. After twelve days, the seeds placed near the routers had not grown. The seeds in the other room were thriving.[96]

Other Voices on Health in this Virtual Season

Leah Morton, MD, doctor of family medicine, New Mexico: *My patients frequently report that their health worsened when they got a cell phone or Wi-Fi, or an antenna or a "smart" meter was installed near their home, school or workplace. They need to drastically reduce their exposure to radiation, but where can they go? Giving up one's own wireless devices is enormously challenging, but it is* possible. *I do not know, however, how anyone can avoid radiation emitted by antennas, neighbors', schools' and businesses' Wi-Fi routers, "smart" meters, fluorescent lights, or other peoples' mobile devices.*

ꕥ

Caroline Adair, 37, California: *I have nearly given up on doctors. First, almost every office has Wi-Fi, fluorescent lights, large TVs in the waiting room, and digitalized equipment and computers in each treatment room. Most doctors*

Association, vol. 63, no. 4 (2013): 459–462.

96 See www.liveleak.com/view?i=cd3_1369428648.

now carry a mobile phone in their breast pocket. Even in an emergency, I would not go to a hospital. Each one is flooded with fluorescent lights, "smart" meters and Wi-Fi; some have rooftop antennas, creating exactly the kind of environment that makes me sick.

❦

Catherine Kleiber, electricalpollution.com, Wisconsin: *In 1996, shortly after graduating from college, my husband and I bought a farm. The following winter, spending more time indoors, I became sick with an illness that just wouldn't lift. I woke feeling unwell. I was only in my early twenties, but I got heart palpitations from going up stairs. I had acid reflux and extremely dry skin. From September until May, my toes kept red, cold and sore. I had chills, low-grade fevers and drenching night sweats. Exertion often left me feeling like I had lactic acid burning in my muscles. Washing dishes, I got lightheaded. After cooking on my electric stove, I felt too sick to eat. I had nerve pain, everywhere.*

After five years, my husband and I learned that we had high frequencies on our wiring, which came from fluorescent lights, electronics, variable speed frequency drives (used by heating systems, milking machines and other common appliances) on our electrical grid.

As an experiment, we turned our circuits off at night. Almost immediately, I woke feeling well rested. The nerve pain and many other symptoms went away. But a week later, I woke full of despair again. I figured that my week of feeling better was a fluke. Then I flipped on a light. It went on, and I realized that my husband had forgotten to turn off the circuits the night before. So, my private "blind" study showed that electrical pollution affects my health.

We installed a dielectric union in the water pipes to prevent electric current from getting onto our water line. We got a gas stove and shut off all non-essential power. Later, when they became available, we installed Graham-Stetzer plug-in filters around the house. I got yet more relief and began to carry them with me for meetings and social gatherings.

After my health improved, my husband and I had two wonderful children. Then, in 2009, our electric company began installing AMR transmitting utility meters in our area. Immediately, the RF levels in our home increased, even though we had no transmitting meter and no near neighbors. In fall 2010, our younger son began waking in the middle of the night, saying that he didn't feel well. Eventually, I noticed that his heart was racing. Over a period of months, as his system wore down, his heartbeat changed from overly fast to slow and irregular, and finally to extremely slow and irregular.

I felt lucky to know that radio-frequency signals can cause cardiac arrhythmias, including in children. To reduce his exposure to RF signals, we disconnected circuits and removed wiring. With each modification, his health improved.

But our utility company installed more transmitting meters around us, and our neighbors used more electronics—which put more high frequency fields on our grid. The electrical pollution at our end-of-the-line home intensified. The radiation coming off of the transformer on our property made fissures on the bark of our sugar maple trees. While asleep, our younger son sweated profusely, and his sweat had a strange odor.

In summer 2011, a mobile cardiac Holter monitor showed that he had 1,500 bradycardia incidents per hour while he slept. A heart beating too slowly is a bradycardia event. A five-year-old boy should not experience them.

To decrease our exposure, we moved into a tent more than a half-mile from any electrical service. Immediately, we noticed improvement in our children's health. While deeply asleep in the tent, our younger son never had more than 200 bradycardia incidents per hour. Once, sleeping back in the house because of broken tent poles, it got so slow that he lost bladder control.

Realizing that neither our public service commission nor our utility company would mitigate the high frequency fields coming into our house on the utility wiring and that we could lose our son, we went off-grid. We installed a gravity flow hot water heating system, a solar system (filtered) and a well pump and sump pumps that operate with direct current, also filtered. We got a propane refrigerator and battery-operated camping lights. We modified our computer so that it runs off of our battery bank, and we only use it when the bank is not charging. For Internet access, we use dial-up. Because the washing machine requires the generator (and its use puts high frequencies on our wiring), everyone gets out of the house at laundry time. We dry our clothes on the line outside or in the basement.

If someone had told us beforehand the lengths to which we would go to be healthy, we would NEVER have believed it.

We're still adjusting to the fact that wireless technologies have made us socially isolated. Our children can't go to school, soccer or gymnastics because these places all have transmitting utility meters and lots of mobile phones in use—and the RF radiation makes our boys sick.

Our seven-year-old often says, "I understand that those devices are convenient, but why would anyone risk their life to make a phone call or watch a video?"

I tell him denial is a powerful force. I tell him I don't really have an answer to his question.

Jennifer Litt, 53, Northeast: *In 2009, when "smart" meters were installed on our gas line, we began to do research and learned that our electric company installed a transmitting AMR meter on our house sometime in 1998, one foot from our infant son's bed. Our son was born in July 1998. I had a difficult labor with Pitocin. He was suctioned and given oxygen. In his first year, he screamed for hours at a time. Was that colic? Was it the result of his difficult birth? Was it irritation from the meter?*

We had been a healthy family, but after 1998, we all had difficulty sleeping. I had nausea, burning and itching with an intermittent rash. My son had heart palpitations and chest pain. We never had Wi-Fi, but my daughter (born in 1990) got severe headaches and sometimes vomited at school when she was exposed to Wi-Fi and "smart" meters.

In 2010, after nine persistent months and a note from our doctor, we got the transmitting meters removed from our house. We can sleep now, and my son's heart palpitations went away.

At school, if my son uses a Wi-Fi-enabled laptop, he gets a headache, his chest hurts, and he feels tingling sensations. So, his teachers let him work without a Wi-Fi-enabled laptop. Still, we need a doctor who can help us and an affordable house with enough space from neighbors so we don't have to absorb radiation from their wireless devices.

In France, mobile phones are banned from primary schools, and advertising of mobile phones that targets children is prohibited.[97] In March 2013, the French National Assembly voted to exercise the Precautionary Principle, protect young children's health and prefer cabled Internet over Wi-Fi in schools.[98]

97 See www.lesondesmobiles.fr/.

98 See www.cnetfrance.fr/news/lesdesputes-ne-veulent-pas-de-wi-fi-dans-les-establissements-scolaires-39788397.htm.

Just How Many Children Use Wireless Devices?

More than 75% of twelve to seventeen-year-olds own mobile phones.[99]

In 2011, Common Sense Media reported, in "Zero to Eight: Children's Media Use in America," that 52% of all children have access to either a smartphone (42%), a video iPod (21%), or an iPad or another tablet device (8%). Ten percent of 0- to one-year-olds, 39% of two- to four-year-olds, and 52% of five- to eight-year-olds have used these newer mobile devices.[100]

A 2011 survey by Elizabeth Englander of 20,000 students in Massachusetts found that 20% of third graders had a cell phone, 40% of fifth graders had one, and 83% of middle schoolers had one.[101]

In a typical day, the average eight- to-ten-year-old spends nearly eight hours with a variety of media; older children and teens spend more than eleven hours per day.[102] If there's a TV in the child's bedroom, these figures increase; and 71% of children and teens report that they have a TV in their bedroom.[103]

A bedroom TV increases a child's risk for obesity, substance use, and exposure to sexual content.[104]

---

99 See http://www.pewinternet.org/2010/04/20/teens-and-mobile-phones/.

100 See www.commonsensemedia.org/research/zero-eight-childrens-media-use-america.

101 E. K. Englander, "Research findings: MARC 2011 survey grades 3–12": http://vcc.bridgew.edu/marc_reports/2.

102 V. Rideout, "Generation M^2: Media in the lives of 8- to 18-year-olds," Kaiser Family Foundation, 2010; www.kaiserfamilyfoundation.files.wordpress.com/2013/01/8010.pdf

103 Ibid.

104 A. E. Staiano et al, "Television, adiposity and cardiometabolic risk in children and adolescents," *American Journal of Preventive Medicine,* vol. 44, no. 1 (2013): 40–47; C. Jackson et al, "A TV in the bedroom: Implications for viewing habits and risk behaviors during early adolescence," *Journal of Broadcasting and Electronic Media,*

Indeed, the media landscape has changed drastically in one generation. Yet, few parents or teachers have rules about media use for the children in their care—rules that limit exposure to EMR or violent content, or rules that prevent or address addiction to media.

In October 2013, the American Academy of Pediatrics (AAP) issued a policy statement, "Managing Media: We Need a Plan." It recommends that parents and pediatricians model "media diets" to help their children learn to be selective and healthy in their consumption of media. In other words, the AAP recommends that parents and pediatricians limit their own media use in order to help children limit their use. The AAP recommends that entertainment screen time be limited to less than one or two hours per day. For children under two, the AAP discourages screen media exposure.

Cellular Antennas on School Grounds and Rooftops

How many cellular antennas have been installed on school grounds and rooftops? What impact do they have on children's long term health? How can we decrease or eliminate cell towers on school campuses?

For now, these questions have no answers.

In September 2006, the Healthy Schools Network (HSN), a national environmental not-for-profit corporation dedicated to assuring every child and school employee an environmentally safe and healthy school, submitted an *amicus curiae* brief

---

vol. 52, no. 3 (2008): 349–367; A. M. Adachi-Mejia et al, "Children with a TV in their bedroom at higher risk for being overweight," *International Journal of Obesity*, vol. 31, no. 44 (2007): 644–651; J. L. Kim et al, "Sexual readiness, household policies and other predictors of adolescents' exposure to sexual content in mainstream entertainment television," *Journal of Media Psychology*, vol. 8, no. 4 (2006): 449–471; E. L. Gruber et al, "Private television viewing, parental supervision, and sexual and substance use risk behaviors in adolescents," *Journal of Adolescent Health*, vol. 36, no. 2 (2005): 107.

to advise the U.S. Supreme Court of the need for enforcement of a court-mandated Environmental Impact Study (EIS) *before* the FCC deployed new Advanced Wireless Services. HSN was "quite concerned that a significant threat to the health of school children and personnel is posed by RF radiation from cell towers placed on or near schools or day centers."

Healthy Schools Network urged the Court to act by the Precautionary Principle. It illuminated that by ignoring the National Environmental Policy Act requirement of an EIS, the FCC risked biological harm to the country's 54 million vulnerable children.[105]

The Court decided not to hear the Healthy Schools Network's case.

In the Environmental Protection Agency's February 8, 2012, draft of *State School Environmental Health Guidelines*, the following "common environmental health issues in K-12 schools" are discussed: routine cleaning and maintenance, mold and moisture, chemicals and environmental contaminants, good ventilation and pests and reducing pesticide use." Health hazards related to magnetic fields from dirty power and RFs from mobile phones, laptops and pads, Wi-Fi, cellular antennas, and "smart" meters are not mentioned.

Parents, Take Note

The American Academy of Pediatrics and Kaiser Permanente warn that too much screen time is associated with children's violent behavior, poor school performance, lower reading scores, sleep pattern disturbances, obesity, and bad habits later in life such as tobacco and alcohol abuse.[106] Kaiser recommends

105 "Brief of Healthy Schools Network, Inc. as *Amicus curiae* in support of Petitioner Maria Gonzales," US Supreme Court, 06–175, 9-5-2006.

106 A-M. Tobin, "Limit screen time for healthier kids" (search at kaiserpermanente.org); V. C. Strasburger and B. J. Wilson, *Children, Adolescents, and the Media,* Thousand Oaks, CA: Sage, 2002, pp. 73ff.

limiting screen time to less than two hours a day for teens, less than one hour a day for children ages three through twelve, and no screen time for children under three. To reduce screen time, Kaiser suggests:

- turning the TV off during meals
- keeping TVs, computers and video game consoles out of kids' bedrooms
- keeping cell phones and iPods out of bedrooms at night
- not using screen time as a reward
- exercising as a family by walking, riding bikes, or playing sports together
- encouraging your children to write a story or create an art project.[107]

⌘

Sandi Maurer, EMFsafetynetwork.org: *Throughout the U.S., schools have begun providing children with wireless computer tablets for learning and testing. New, stronger routers are being installed in classrooms. The Los Angeles Unified School District is issuing wireless iPads, even to elementary-aged students. This push for computers in the classroom is part of Common Core State Standards, the new federal curriculum. It eliminates community-based planning. It brings computer testing into schools and gives the government a new tool to track and profile children.*

Few parents (and educators) are well informed about the issues. For example, in the Fall of 2013, a Sebastopol, California, School Board received funding to upgrade their computer system. As Director of the EMF Safety Network and a parent, I presented the School Board with expert science and medical warnings that RF radiation emitted by routers and wireless computers can cause learning, concentration, memory and many other serious health problems.

107 A-M. Tobin, ibid.

I asked the Board to apply the Precautionary Principle and create a hard-wired computer lab that would provide safer, faster and more secure Internet access, since all children are at risk in a wireless environment. Children who already experience headaches, heart palpitations, seizures, EMF sensitivity and/or who have medical implants are at even greater risk. Such children may be isolated from peers when computers are used; or school may become inaccessible to them.

Dozens of other parents and teachers signed a letter stating, "Key to the (children's) professional success, social integration and economic sustainability, and therefore their health, will be their ability to navigate the world of technology." These well-intentioned parents urged the school board to invest "in computer infrastructure that is portable, wireless and cost effective."

The Board approved the wireless plan.

iPad Health Risks

In its users' manual, Apple warns iPad users about the device's health risks, including headaches, blackouts, seizures, convulsion, eye or muscle twitching, loss of awareness, involuntary movement, or disorientation.

The Apple Support Forum (discussions.apple.com/) posts consumer complaints such as:

> *"Is it just me or does someone else also feel dizzy or nausea after using iPad for a while?"*

> *"I looove the iPad, but I don't think I can keep it as I get nausea and feel a bit dizzy just using it for a few minutes."*

> *"Just today finished series of tests...echocardiogram, brain scan, ultrasound on carotid artery, the works...to diagnose dizziness, and even one fainting episode...since Xmas. Guess what I got for Christmas...iPad..."*

7

Other Dangers from Wireless Devices

Let me state again that electronic technologies have created profound benefits in nearly every aspect of human life. However, because we have not sufficiently tested or regulated new devices and equipment nor their use in combination, we have also created great hazards. Here are other issues that deserve more attention than this book provides.

Energy and Natural Resources

Because of their huge servers (which store data and access apps that let people share music or photos via the Internet for cloud computing), companies like Amazon, Apple, and Microsoft use vast amounts of electric power. In "How Green Is Your Cloud?" Greenpeace Senior Policy Analyst Gary Cook describes data centers so big that they are visible from space and require as much energy as it takes to power 250,000 European homes. Greenpeace also explains that if the cloud were its own country, it would rank fifth in the world in energy consumption.

In the September 23, 2012, *NY Times*, James Glanz, in the article "Power, Pollution and the Internet: Industry Wastes Vast Amounts of Electricity, Belying Image," reported that worldwide, data centers roughly require the equivalent of the output of thirty nuclear power plants.

Individual wireless devices also hog energy and contribute to our environment's degradation. A mobile phone uses three times as much energy as a landline. One search on Google requires as much energy as a 100 watt bulb uses to burn for six minutes.[1]

In *Consuming the Congo: War and Conflict Minerals in the World's Deadliest Place*, Peter Eichstaedt describes how mining in Congo for coltan, a mineral necessary for cell phones, has contributed to mass rapes and more loss of life than any other single situation since World War II.

Worker Safety and Violation of Radiation Limits

In March 2013, the *EMR Policy Institute (EMRPI)* launched "Americans Beware," a campaign to alert workers and families about nationwide violations of FCC radiation limits. EMRPI tested industry-operated antenna sites in 23 states and found them in gross violation (up to and in excess of 600%) of the FCC's public exposure rates. This means, for example, that hundreds of thousands of people who work on rooftops and cannot avoid standing near antennas (that do not have adequately posted warnings or barriers) are exposed to radiation beyond FCC limits. The FCC has not levied a single fine against a wireless carrier for exceeding these limits. The EMRPI called on Congress to hold the FCC accountable, to inform Americans about their risk of unlawful exposure to radiation—and their right to protection from such exposure.[2]

On May 22, 2012, PBS Frontline News reported, in "Cell Tower Deaths" that "independent contractors who are building and servicing America's cellular infrastructure are ten times more likely than the average construction worker to die on the job." WirelessEstimator.com notes that "complex layers

1 E. Pariser, *The Filter Bubble: What the Internet is Hiding from You*, New York: Penguin, 2011.

2 Search youtube.com: "Wireless Industry Safety Failure," part 1.

of subcontracting insulate the carriers against liability, despite the fact that they set the aggressive schedule that can force subcontractors to cut corners in order to meet deadlines, and those ambitious time frames may be one of the reasons why workers are dying."

Fires Caused by Telecom Equipment and "Smart" Meters

On April 26, 2009, ABC News confirmed that the Malibu, California fires were caused by utility poles "overburdened by new cellular phone gear." Power poles that should have withstood winds of 92 mph snapped in 50 mph winds due to "heavy wind catching cables and antennas."

In Pennsylvania, installation of "smart" meters caused twenty-six fires and millions of dollars in damages. As a result, in August 2012, PECO (Pennsylvania's electric utility) suspended further installation.

Hacking and Privacy

According to Washington University law professor Neil M. Richards, laws protecting individuals' intellectual privacy have not kept up with technology. For example, while librarians are bound by statutes and ethics not to disclose patrons' reading selections, corporations like Apple, Amazon, and Barnes & Noble are guided by privacy policies they write themselves.[3] Subscribers may not realize that their mobile phones essentially function as tracking devices. Many employers, including Harvard University, routinely scan their employees' email.[4]

Because wireless devices can easily be hacked, personal information is regularly stolen, threatening peoples' finances and entire lives. The annual cost of identity theft alone is thought to

3 A. Sultan, "Online, your reading habits are an open book," *St. Louis Post-Dispatch*, 9-24-2012.

4 See more at the Electronic Frontier Foundation, which defends rights in the digital world; www.eff.org.

be $5 billion for consumers and $50 billion for companies. A.M. Best, a full-service credit rating organization, warned the insurance industry on February 14, 2013 (ambest.com), about data breaches, "risks associated with long-term use of cell phones" and "dangers to the estimated 250,000 workers who come in close contact with cell phone antennas."

In a 2012 *Washington Post* series, "The Threat in Cyberspace," reporters observed that "to succeed in addressing risks in the digital universe, global leaders must understand one of the most complex, human-made creations on Earth: cyberspace."[5]

On April 12, 2012, Marketwatch.com, an investor site, hacking expert David Chalk said that because of risk of cyber attack to the "smart" grid, there is a "100% certainty of catastrophic failure of the energy grid within three years. This could actually be worse than a nuclear war, because it would happen everywhere. How governments and utilities are blindly merging the power grid with the Internet, and effectively without any protection, is insanity at its finest." Chalk speaks in the documentary, "Take Back Your Power," at thepowerfilm.org.

The Loss of Libraries and History

In this virtual season, computers and programs become obsolete almost immediately. For example, the Library of Congress's oral history interviews with Vietnam vets are on disks that only one computer can read, and *very* few people know how to repair it.

Archivists have explained to me that if someone alters a paper document, anyone can *see* the change. And paper documents can't easily be disposed. If documents are only digitalized, then anyone can change them—and revise history—just by changing the font. A digital document can be deleted with a keystroke.

5 See www.washingtonpost.com/investigations/health-care-sector-vulnerable-to-hackers-researchers-say/2012/12/25/left.

Also, because few people have kept paper records in the last twenty years, this period of history is not well recorded.

Many textbooks are now only available online, which disables people who can't use a computer because of financial or physical limitations. Further, e-textbooks typically stop being available to students once their course is over. This makes the fundamental information that people learn in school inaccessible after just a few months.

Since medical journals cost between six and twelve hundred dollars per year, *and* they require storage space, many hospitals have eliminated their libraries. One corporate chain might spend ten thousand dollars for staff in ten hospitals to access two hundred and fifty digitalized medical journals. This is much less expensive than paper journals and requires no storage space. With a hand-held device, a doctor can access medical studies online, read an abstract at a patient's bedside and research treatment options and dosage amounts without waiting. Historically, research has meant leafing through shelves, comparing books and discussing issues with other researchers. *How does digital research change what gets discovered?*

Psychological Issues

In *Virtually You: The Dangerous Powers of the E-Personality*, psychiatrist Elias Aboujaoude describes how participating in the Internet allows us to act with exaggerated confidence and sexiness, making us impatient, unfocused, and urge-driven.

Distracted Drivers and Walkers

According to the National Highway Traffic Safety Administration, distracted drivers killed more than 3,300 people in the U.S. in 2011, with another 387,000 people hurt. Apparently, even talking on a hands-free device, including a voice-to-text system, leaves a driver with less brainpower for driving. In 2005,

Australian researchers found that drivers using hands-free and hand-held cell phones were four times as likely to crash as those not on a phone.[6] On August 27, 2013, the Superior Court of New Jersey ruled that texters can be held responsible in civil court for distracting a driver if they have "special reason to know...from prior texting experience...that the recipient will view the text while driving." In such cases, "the sender has breached a duty of care to the public by distracting the driver."[7]

A nationwide study by Ohio State University researchers published in the August 2013 issue of *Accident Analysis and Prevention* estimates that more than 1,500 pedestrians were treated in emergency rooms in 2010 for injuries related to using a cell phone while walking. Jack Nasar, the study's coauthor, thinks that these numbers are "much lower than what is really happening." He said that he wouldn't be surprised if this number doubles between 2010 and 2015. Young adults aged twenty-one to twenty-five are most likely to be injured by distracted walking, followed by sixteen- to twenty-year-olds.

"Parents already teach their children to look both ways when crossing the street. They should also teach them," Nasar cautioned, "to put away their cell phone when walking, particularly when crossing a street."

Flight Safety

For more than a decade, pilots and scientific studies have reported that passengers' mobile devices interfere with airplane equipment. In some cases, one cell phone's signals can blot out global-positioning satellites and render a plane's GPS receivers useless. As our aviation system transitions to satellite-based navigation, the risk of harmful interference from passengers'

6 J. Hecht, "Hands-free tools make driving more dangerous," *The Associated Press*, 8-1-2013.

7 M. Pearce, "Court paves way for blame of texters who distract drivers," *LA Times*, 8-30-2013.

phones and pads increases. Meanwhile, nearly half of all passengers want to use their devices during all phases of flight.[8]

If one phone can create "harmful interference" with a GPS, what could it do to a child's brain?

Worker Safety

Routinely now, electrical workers and workers in other trades may be exposed to RF radiation from antennas without knowing that they are being exposed or how to protect themselves. In his September 11, 2013, Comment to the FCC about radiofrequency exposure limits and policies, Edwin D. Hill, International President of the International Brotherhood of Electrical Workers (IBEW) stated, "we believe that many of our members have been exposed to levels of RF radiation in excess of the FCC limits."

"When there is a hazard," Mr. Hill further states, "the hazard creator has a duty to warn others against the hazard." He suggests that telecom companies that are licensed to deploy transmitting antennas should be responsible for ensuring that IBEW members "know the unique physical boundaries at every work location so as not to exceed the referenced RF exposure limits." At present, telecom companies are not required to post signs that inform workers that an antenna (which may be disguised or in a chimney) is nearby. A. M. Best Company estimates that 250,000 workers come into close contact with cellular antennas every year. It warns other insurers that at close range, cellular antennas act "essentially as open microwave ovens;" and that exposed workers' health effects "can include eye damage, sterility and cognitive impairments."[9]

---

8 A. Levin, "'Off' button key to pilot interference reports," *Bloomberg News*, 5-16-2013.

9 "Emerging Technologies Pose Significant Risks with Possible Long-Tail Losses," *Best's Briefing*, 2-14-2013.

Liability

Underwriters A.M. Best and Lloyds of London advise insurance companies not to ensure against damages to health caused by wireless devices, including cellular antennas. Swiss RE rates electromagnetic fields (EMF) higher than any other emerging risk.[10]

A.M. Best notes that "the continued exponential growth of cellular towers will significantly increase exposure to these workers and others."[11]

In the event that damages to health caused by antennas, mobile phones or "smart" meters are proven in court, no corporation will be insured (beyond self-insurance) to pay for such damages.

Continuing Developments

According to "Wireless Technologies and the National Information Infrastructure," issued by the U.S. Congress' Office of Technology Assessment in July 1995, "New technologies will continue to be introduced that cannot be tested in all real-world situations. A recent example: the operator's manual for European-model BMW automobiles advises owners not to use a digital (GSM) cellular telephone while driving the car, because it may interfere with the car's electrical system and lead to permanent deployment of the airbags."

With the Obama administration's support, Light Squared, a telecom company, aimed to beam 4G WiMax to 97% of the U.S. by 2018. Because Light Squared's signals interfere with GPS networks, this program has been set back.[12]

---

10 See http://mieuxprevenir.blogspot.com/2011/12/swiss-re-will-not-re-insure-mobile.html.

11 "Emerging Technologies Pose Significant Risks with Possible Long-Tail Losses," *Best's Briefing*, Feb.14, 2013.

12 See commlawblog.com/2012/02/articles/cellular/federal-gps-sers-nix-lightsquared/index.html.

In 2009, AT&T petitioned the FCC with a request to abandon their landline equipment because maintenance costs are so high.

In January, 2014, James Porter, Director of Telecommunications for the Vermont Department of Public Service, suggested in his report to the state legislature, "Costs and Profitability of Vermont's Incumbent Telecommunications Carriers" that most Vermonters are happy with fast-tracking permits for wireless services. He questioned how long state regulators can require phone companies to maintain landlines that are no longer profitable. Demand for landlines is down in populated areas (where maintenance is less expensive), and maintaining service in sparsely populated areas (where landlines are more popular) is expensive. In response to Mr. Porter's questions, Matt Levin, a lobbyist with Vermonters for a Clean Environment, wondered how regulators will ensure that everyone who wants (or needs) a landline will have one. "Who will pay to maintain landline infrastructure," Levin asked, "when only a small percentage of our population uses landlines? And what will we do in twenty years if we decide that mobile phones are bad for our health, we need landlines, and our landline infrastructure has disappeared?"

8

Rules and Regulations that Frame Us

The existing FCC and international limits do not do enough to protect people, especially children, from daily exposures to electromagnetic fields and radio frequency radiation. The existing safety limits did not anticipate these new kinds of technologies affecting the health of people living with and using wireless devices on a daily basis. (Biological) effects are now widely reported to occur at exposure levels significantly below most current national and international limits.

David O. Carpenter, MD, Coeditor of *The BioInitiative Report* Director of the Institute for Health and the Environment, SUNY, Albany

As people invented wheels, carts, then horse-drawn buggies, they noticed the need for measures that kept travelers and bystanders safe. For examples, to stop a horse pulling a carriage, the driver needs a way to signal the horse to halt, and a breaking system for the buggy's wheels. Motorized vehicles need windshield wipers, seat belts, children's seats, and air bags. We paved roads, set speed limits, created intersections with stop signs and stop lights. For the most part, these protective measures kept pace with new vehicles.

A Summary of the Rules for Our Electric Grid and Telecommunications

It's this simple: our rules and regulations for electricity, electronics, transmission antennas, and wireless devices serve engineering needs. Our laws do not consider these technologies' impacts on public health or the environment—except, in some cases, to make such consideration a liability.

Briefly, here are our federal regulations around electricity, electronics, transmitters, wireless devices and health:

- No federal agency regulates our 60 Hz electrical grid, including "smart" installations.
- The FCC defines "harmful interference" as anything that interferes with existing radio, TV, or Internet broadcasts. No agency defines "biological harm" from transformers or broadcasting equipment. No agency has funding to regulate magnetic fields or RF fields that have the potential to harm health or wildlife.
- Section 704 of the Telecommunications Act of 1996 states that no health or environmental concern can interfere with the placement of telecom equipment.
- In August 2013, the FCC reclassified the outer part of the ear as an extremity, meaning that mobile devices near it are allowed a Specific Absorption Rate (SAR) of 4.0 W/kg, significantly higher than the 1.6 W/kg allowed for non-extremities such as the head and trunk.
- No regulations address the effects of magnetic fields or RFs on special populations, including pregnant women, children, people with medical implants, or the infirm.
- Environmental Impact Studies (EISs), required by the National Environmental Policy Administration (NEPA), have not been honored when installing cellular antennas or other transmitters on or near schools or in sensitive habits.

FCC Regulations

Since we began generating and delivering electricity throughout the U.S. in the early 1900s, no federal agency has regulated our electrical grid, including "smart" installations. The FCC regulates non-government devices that operate above 9 kHz and below 300 GHz. The National Telecommunications and Information Agency (NTIA) regulates government equipment. Power lines operate below 9 kHz. Metal detectors (like those at airports) operate above 300 GHz. In other words, no federal agency regulates power lines or metal detectors.

In 1934, Congress authorized the FCC to regulate electronic devices and systems that have the potential to interfere with existing broadcasts. This means that when a manufacturer wants to market a new device, it must prove to the FCC that the new product will not interfere with existing radio, TV, or (now) Internet broadcasts. Said another way, the FCC recognizes that some frequencies can harm *electronics*, and that some devices create "harmful interference" with existing broadcasts. No agency recognizes that magnetic or RF fields can cause *biological* harm.

According to the *BioInitiative Report*, the FCC's regulations allow exposure to electromagnetic radiation that is at least one thousand times higher than what the BioInitiative scientists find is safe for public health.[1]

In 1996, the FCC established an allowable SAR for mobile devices. Again, these regulations are based on engineering needs, and do not consider biological effects.

FDA Regulations

In 1971, more than a decade after a cardiac pacemaker was first implanted in a person and patients had reported interference

1 See www.BioInitiative.org; it recommends keeping exposure levels below 1,000 u µW/m2. The Seletun Statement recommends keeping exposure levels below 1,700 µW/m2. FCC exposure limit levels for cell phone radiation are 6 to 10 million µW/m2.

between their implants and microwave ovens, the Food and Drug Administration (FDA) began requiring microwave oven owners to post a notice that an oven is nearby, since its electromagnetic signals can interfere with a pacemaker's.

In 1970, the FDA's Bureau of Radiological Health (now the Center for Devices and Radiological Health) determined that after purchase, a microwave oven's specific absorption rate (SAR) should not exceed five mW per square centimeter at any point, five centimeters or more from the oven's external surface.[2] For cell phones, as of August 2013, the FCC's SAR limit is 4.0 W/kg for extremities (including the earlobe) within 1 gram of tissue, significantly more than microwave ovens are allowed.

In the U.S., the Institute of Electrical and Electronics Engineers (IEEE) and the National Council for Radiation Protection and Measurements develop recommendations for safety standards that are then regulated by the FCC. Each of these agencies is concerned with engineering, not health. Indeed, in 2003, IEEE's Eleanor Adair, chair of the International Committee on Electromagnetic Safety, wrote that it is "important that safety standards be rational and *avoid excessive safety margins*."[3]

No agency has determined SAR limits for pregnant women, children, or people with medical implants. No agency studies the health or behavior of children born to parents who no longer have landlines.

The FDA still has the authority to regulate any device that emits radiation, including color TVs, baby monitors, mobile phones, and Wi-Fi; but Congress has not given it the funding to do so. Similarly, the Environmental Protection Agency (EPA)

2 See www.accessdata.fda.gov/scripts/cdrh/cfdocs/cfcfr/CFRSearch.cfm?fr=1030.10.

3 J. M. Osepchuk and R. C. Petersen, "Historical review of RF exposure standards and the International Committee on Electromagnetic Safety (ICES)," *Bioelectromagnetic Supplement*, suppl. 6 (2003): 7–16 (emphasis added).

has the authority to regulate human-made electromagnetic radiation in our environment; but in the 1980s, Congress took away all funding for it to do so.

The Telecommunications Act of 1996

In 1996, President Clinton signed the Telecommunications Act (the TCA) into law. As explained earlier, Section 704 of the TCA prohibits municipal and state legislators from refusing to permit installation of telecom equipment based on health or environmental concerns. If the corporation believes that your city councilors took health into account when denying them a permit, then the telecom corporation can sue your city.

If your city council takes too much time to process a telecom corporation's application to install equipment, then the corporation can sue your city.

According to the TCA, your town can only refuse to permit installation of wireless equipment if it does not like how an antenna *looks* or if the equipment's presence or appearance decreases property values.

Telecommunications in Court

How have these rules and regulations affected real people and wildlife? How have they played out in court?

In the late '90s, a telecom company installed cellular antennas on a radio tower near Burlington, Vermont. The antennas' signals interfered with a nearby veterinarian's equipment, which monitored animals' vital signs during surgery. The interference prevented this vet from performing surgery safely. Citizens in her town sued, aiming for the antennas to be mitigated or moved to another location. In 2000, the U.S. Second Circuit judges ruled that if a telecom company has received an FCC license to operate, then nearby residents, organizations and businesses must accept blanket interference. The citizens appealed the case to the U.S. Supreme Court, but the court chose not to take the case. The veterinarian moved her practice.

When the Connecticut Siting Council granted Cellco (Verizon) a permit to install a cell tower near a sensitive bird habitat without first requiring the company to conduct an environmental impact study, citizen Dina Jaeger urged the Council to shift the tower site to avoid harming the area's migratory birds. The Council rejected her arguments, including scientific studies, on the ground that the Telecom Act of 1996 preempted the Migratory Bird Treaty and barred any agency action. Ms. Jaeger petitioned the U.S. Supreme Court to direct Connecticut and other states to obey international migratory bird treaties designed to protect birds by outlawing the placement of cell towers in flyways, nesting areas, and habitats. On June 28, 2011, the Supreme Court announced its refusal to hear the case.

In 2012, a telecom company proposed installing 4G WiMax via a Distributed Antenna System (DAS) on existing utility poles near a sensitive California habitat. To install a new cell tower near a sensitive habitat, a telecom company must first prepare a review of the installation's environmental impact for the National Environmental Policy Administration (NEPA). This requirement is exempted for installations on existing poles.

While nearby residents oppose installing the DAS, the shot-clock rule, adopted by the FCC in 2009, requires that municipalities must grant or deny permits for telecom antennas within 90 days for co-locations, and 150 days for new equipment. If the municipality does not make a final decision on the company's request within 90 or 150 days, then installation of the equipment is automatically approved. Because these short time periods do not allow for local requirements like adequate public notice, a public hearing or an appeals procedure, telecom companies can effectively install antennas as they please—without respect for local concerns—including in sensitive habitats.

The City of Arlington, Texas requested that the U.S. Court of Appeals for the Fifth Circuit invalidate the shot-clock rule; but the Court of Appeals upheld it. The Supreme Court agreed to hear the case. Los Angeles, San Antonio, and several other municipalities joined Arlington's challenge of the FCC ruling. AT&T, Verizon, T-Mobile and the Personal Communications Infrastructure Association-Wireless Infrastructure Association submitted briefs in support of the FCC's shot-clock rule. In May, 2013, the Supreme Court voted in favor of the FCC ruling and the telecom companies.

In 2010, an electrically sensitive man who is disabled by signals from cellular antennas, filed a suit against the City of Santa Fe, New Mexico and AT&T, claiming that according to the Americans with Disabilities Act (the ADA) and the Fourteenth Amendment, the installation of telecom equipment violates his rights. At AT&T's request, the case was transferred from a state court to a federal court, where a judge ruled that the Telecommunications Act preempts the ADA—even though the ADA was enacted in 1991, and the TCA stated, when it passed in 1996, that all previous Acts of Congress must be obeyed. The federal judge ruled that since a more specifically worded statute (like the TCA) takes precedent over a statute that is more generally worded (like the ADA), the Telecom Act preempts the ADA. He outlined that the best recourse for people who are disabled by telecom radiation is to get Congress to revise Section 704 of the TCA. In October 2012, the Court of Appeals ruled that the case should not have been transferred to federal court and returned it to the New Mexico court. In October 2013, the electrically sensitive man asked for a *writ of mandamus*, a court order that would require the City of Santa Fe to enforce its own laws—and require a new, public hearing for any intensification of cell tower emissions. At this writing, the decision awaits.

Many other lawsuits about wireless devices are now making their way through the courts. In June 2013, the law firms of David Kyle and Paul Overett filed a class action lawsuit against California's PG&E and SC Edison because of "smart" meters' health effects (including headaches, loss of energy, ringing in the ears, cancer, heart attacks, and medical implant interference). Citizens in Naperville, Illinois and in Maine are also fighting "smart" meters. A case in Portland, Oregon, involves the effects of Wi-Fi on a diabetic child in a public school.

Other Challenges to Our Laws

While nearly every place in the U.S. has become chronically exposed to radio-frequency fields from military and police radar, Wi-Fi, mobile devices, cellular antennas, "smart" meters, and other transmitters, some citizens have challenged our federal rules and regulations. Here are their stories:

ꕥ

Jo-Tina DiGennaro: *I live in Bayville, NY, a small town on Long Island. Starting about 1992, without proper notice to nearby residents, our water tower began to house antennas. By 2009, it had accumulated nearly sixty antennas. Our elementary school's property line is fifty feet from our water tower. Between 2000 and 2007, four children in our village were diagnosed with leukemia; another child was diagnosed with brain cancer. Three of these five children died. At one point, seven of the school's twenty-one staff members had some form of cancer. For a small village, this is a very high incidence of childhood leukemia and cancer.*

Did the antennas cause this? Did the antennas' put high frequencies on school's wiring? Did the equipment that operates the antennas put electrical currents in the water lines?

We don't know. But we who live near the antennas and who have children and grandchildren at the school are very concerned.

In public and private meetings, our mayor at the time repeatedly stated that the belief that the antennas endanger our children is completely unfounded. After a vote by the town's trustees (five yes, two no) to install more antennas for police equipment on the water tower, several residents became agitated. When a man (who can hear the antennas buzz from his front step and whose baby was nine months old at the time) began to express his concerns, he was not asked to reserve his comments until later. A police officer escorted him out of the building.

Because we want the path of least regret, many of us in Bayville, want the antennas moved. Because of the Telecom Act, we could not speak freely with our town officials or question whether the antennas contribute to our health problems.

Our water tower sits on land that was donated to the town with the condition that the land could never be used for commercial purposes. The deed also states that nothing on this land could be deemed dangerous, offensive or obnoxious to anyone within one mile of the site. Since leasing space on the water tower provides financial gain for the Village of Bayville and for the telecom companies, and since many of us find the telecom equipment on the water tower dangerous, we sued the Village and the telecom companies involved to move the antennas.

A lower court ruled against us. We wanted to pursue the matter to a higher court, but we ran out of money. The five telecom companies involved had money to continue as long as necessary.

Clearly, The 1996 Telecommunications Act protects the telecom corporations. It gives common people no protection.

Meanwhile, I hear more people wanting better reception and wider coverage for their devices than I hear people concerned about the health effects of telecom equipment. Around the country, water towers and other structures are covered with antennas. Radiation levels around these towers can exceed FCC guidelines, which are one thousand times higher than what the BioInitiative Report *researchers consider safe. So I worry—about people who live near antennas, for children who attend school near them and for workers who maintain water towers.*

ꕥ

Deb Carney, attorney: *When television and radio towers first went up on Lookout Mountain in Golden, Colorado, many of the area's residents thought they were ugly. We did not think they could be dangerous. We believed that governmental regulations protected us. After resident scientists, doctors, lawyers and engineers donated thousands of hours to researching antennas' effects on health, we learned that we were* not *protected.*

We learned that in Ukraine, an agency equivalent to the FCC deals with the technical aspects of transmitting signals. An additional agency serves to protect peoples' health. In the U.S., we have no such agency.

With funding from the National Institute of Health, scientists from two universities took blood samples from 300 residents. We learned that as our exposure to radiation increased, so did our white blood counts. Even at radiation levels one hundred times less than what the FCC allows, the scientists found biological effects in our blood samples; and every resident near Lookout Mountain with a brain tumor lived in direct line of sight to the TV/FM towers. The scientists published their findings.[4] *In 1999, the University of Colorado's Department of Radiation Oncology wrote, "Without proper scientific data, we consider it unconscionable to expose the people of Jefferson County to these levels of radiation."*

For eight years, the Golden area's citizens effectively prevented a group of television stations from building a new, 730-foot tower on Lookout Mountain designed to broadcast digital signals to the entire Denver area. Golden area residents and officials feared that an increase in electromagnetic radiation would harm our health, scar the mountain and create electrical interference in nearby homes and businesses. We collected 3,000 signatures from people who did not want a new tower installed.

In 2006, the TV stations hired Wiley Rein & Fielding, a lobbying group that "maintain(s) ongoing professional relationships with the highest Executive Branch officials and key Republican and Democratic members of Congress."

On Saturday, December 9, 2006, 2:09 a.m., a "noncontroversial" bill was "hotlined" through the Senate (and later the House) with no hearing or debate. The bill preempts local zoning control over towers on Lookout Mountain. On December 22, President Bush signed the bill into law. If this could happen to Golden, it can happen anywhere.

ꕤ

Jeff Stone: *I work in a small city's planning and land use department. Recently, a telecom company proposed installing an antenna in a church steeple here. The church houses a nursery school. Parents do not want the antenna installed. To keep*

---

4 J. B. Burch et al, "Radio frequency nonionizing radiation in a community exposed to radio and television broadcasting," *Environmental Health Perspectives,* vol. 114, no. 2 (2006): 248–253; J. S. Reif et al, "Human responses to residential RF exposure: Final report," *Environmental Health Perspectives,* 8.23.05.

their church solvent, board members want the income they'll get from renting the steeple to the telecom company.

As a public servant whose job is to uphold land use codes, my choice is between permitting the antenna and a lawsuit against my city from the telecom company for non-compliance, a lawsuit that they will surely win. Furthermore, my town does not have resources for a court battle.

As I see it, concerned citizens need to educate their neighbors before *any telecom company offers to lease space for antennas from a property owner—and to petition Congress to revise Section 704 of The Telecom Act so that every community can determine its own setback policies for antennas.*

⌘

Gary Olhoeft, PhD, geophysicist and electrical engineer, professor emeritus, Colorado School of Mines: *Despite the fact that ten percent of Americans (more than twenty-five million people) have a medical implant, no agency studies their experience around wireless devices. Many of these people may find their implant malfunctioning (including shutting off) if they board an airplane, share an elevator with a mobile phone user, or step through a security door at a library or a mall. No agency studies the interference that may occur between devices when a cochlear implant is installed in a person who already has a deep brain stimulator and a pacemaker.*

We need to broaden public awareness about the vulnerability of people with medical implants. We also need regulation that will limit electromagnetic emissions. We need to create limits around "second-hand" exposure to electromagnetic radiation since, for example, being in a metal-walled elevator with a person who is using a mobile phone can be especially hazardous for people with implants. At a minimum, stores and other places with security and Wi-Fi devices (now often not visible but hidden behind walls) should post warnings that a potential hazard exists for people with implanted medical devices and radio-frequency sickness.

Such warnings could be modeled after those the FDA began requiring of microwave oven manufacturers in the 1970s. They alerted people with cardiac pacemakers that the oven could leak radiation and create a potential hazard. The FDA still regulates microwave ovens, and most of them leak less radiation than most cell phones. All mobile phones are currently allowed to leak higher SARs than microwave ovens.[5]

ꕥ

Sandra Chianfoni, www.sandaura.wordpress.com, Massachusetts: *In 1999, I bought a house in a rural town of 900 people. Since fall 2006, my family and I have heard a constant, disturbing noise in every room. Outside, we cannot hear birds or the wind without this buzz. I've tried expensive headphones and earplugs, but the noise penetrates them. To sleep, we keep fans on, which helps to mask the noise. Often, I turn on the radio—or the buzz will envelop me. To read on a winter day, I sit with a fan near my head. I cannot find silence. My family and I have not had proper sleep in seven years.*

After a year of thinking something was wrong with our house, we hired a power quality engineer. On our wires, he found a constant harmonic distortion of 60 Hz AC power—double the harmonics allowed by the IEEE. We then retained a certified forensic audio engineer, who analyzed recordings taken at my home, four miles away, and during a power outage throughout our town. This engineer determined that the constant noise measures at 217 Hz in the 250 Hz narrow octave band. It's a "pure tone frequency," a bioactive, noxious, toxic pollutant. As

5 Professor Olhoeft speaks on "Electromagnetic Interference and Medical Implants"; at www.youtube/com/results?search_query=olhoeft&sm#12.

part of the "smart" grid, utility companies use this frequency to communicate data, even during power outages.

Are these the source of the buzz I hear?

In 1972, the EPA set exposure limits on pure tones to protect workers from their negative health effects. Based on these regulations, which the Massachusetts Department of Environmental Protection (DEP) adopted in 1990, I filed complaints with DEP, the state's public utility regulatory agency, and the Department of Public Health, since the pure-tone levels at my house are illegal, since I cannot sleep properly, and since the power surging from the "smart" grid causes high levels of electrical pollution on my electrical system.

The Massachusetts DEP recognizes that extremely low frequencies (ELFs)—such as those transmitted by the pure tone—affect health, but it did not take action with my complaint. The regulatory agency wanted me *to tell* them *the source of the noise. They would not involve the FCC or interview the engineers I'd hired. Instead, they closed my case.*

The case needs to reopen for the whole country. Our electrical grid now serves as a continuous antenna. Wherever the global "smart" grid is turned on, it delivers noxious pure tones into private and public spaces. Wind turbines also emit disturbing noise. Routinely now, I hear from people all over the world who have become agitated, unable to sleep, afraid to buy a home (where the pure tone might become audible), and even suicidal because of this buzz. It makes no sense for individuals to fight it. Until regulatory agencies implement protections, we will all be subject to a festering noise.

⌘

Josh Hart, MSc., StopSmartMeters.org, California: *The "smart" transmitting meters that utility companies have installed around the country pose numerous, significant dangers. Traditional* *analog meters had no electronic components, but digital transmitting "smart" meters run on switch-mode power supplies. They pulse microwaves that travel into homes, schools, hospitals and office buildings that use electricity.*

Supposedly, "smart" meters are designed to help us save energy. However, after Pacific Gas & Electric (one of the largest U.S. utilities) spent billions of ratepayer dollars to install networked meters and data storage facilities, the company's 2010 Program Year Demand Response and Energy Conservation Annual Report *revealed* zero *energy saved.*

StopSmartMeters.org has received more than 1,000 reports from people with rashes, headaches, nausea, dizziness, ringing in the ears, insomnia, bloody noses, heat sensations and much more after a transmitting meter was installed on their home. The California Public Utilities Commission has received more than ten thousand complaints.

Around the world, fires started by "smart" meters are reported nearly every day. EmfSafetyNetwork.org tracks these fires and explosions. People have died as a result of some fires; others have become homeless. Are the fires caused by shoddy installation? By installation on a house whose wiring is not compatible with the meter? We need independent investigations to answer these questions. Meanwhile, insurance companies will not insure against installations of transmitting meters since the socket onto which a meter is attached is considered the property owner's property.

"Smart" meters infringe on peoples' privacy. They reveal daily schedules by providing fine-grain data about customers' use of electricity, gas and water. The information can identify a ratepayer's daily habits. In California and other states, the data is being sold to third parties without ratepayers' consent.

In response to campaigns to prevent the installation of more transmitting meters, the industry created "opt-out" programs, which often charge consumers to keep or restore analog meters. We do not support opt-outs: if a meter is dangerous, and evidence shows that these digital, transmitting meters are indeed dangerous, then no one should be exposed to them. Opt-outs discriminate against people with limited income; and anyone with multiple meters in their neighborhood has to contend with meters' emissions whether or not they pay for an opt-out.

No law states that everyone must have a transmitting meter on their property. People have a right to reject something dangerous, to refuse radiation-emitting, surveillance devices on our homes and schools.

With our current structure, investor-owned utilities take money from ratepayers and distribute profits to shareholders. This presents a crisis and an opportunity for people who need safe delivery of electricity, gas and water. Digital meters must be recalled. We need to make safety, health and quality of life our priorities—and to find real ways to cut our carbon emissions, household by household, community by community.

The Federal Record on Health and RF Field Exposure

While common citizens have fought to protect their homes, schools, and neighborhoods from EMR, the Electromagnetic Radiation Policy Institute (EMRPI) has commented to agencies including the Department of Justice (DOJ), FCC, FDA, Government Accountability Office (GAO), National Academies of Science (NAS), National Institute for Occupational Safety and Health (NIOSH) and the National Telecommunications Information Agency (NTIA) about the health effects of exposure to radio-frequency fields. EMRPI has challenged several cases in the U.S. Circuit Courts of Appeals. It has also filed three petitions for certiorari with the U.S. Supreme Court; but none were accepted (emrpolicy.org/litigation/case_law/index.htm).

In response to EMRPI's challenges, the FCC has repeatedly told Congress and the federal courts that it does not have expertise in RF field exposure health issues. Here is the federal record on health policy and RF field exposure, compiled by EMRPI President Janet Newton:

1995

The U.S. Congress Office of Technology Assessment issued a report, "Wireless Technologies and the National Information Infrastructure." It states that "unintended effects of radio waves" that involve "compatibility problems . . . can, for the most part, be solved either by shielding devices, keeping radio waves away from people and sensitive equipment, or changing the modulation scheme emitting devices used. However, with widespread deployment of small radio devices with complex operating characteristics, it is possible that at some point there will be interference leading to a system failure. Because of the large number of devices, the variety of ways they are used, and the complexity of the possible interactions, it is unlikely that every combination can be tested and potential problems anticipated."

1999

In 1997, the FCC adopted exposure level standards set by the RF Exposure Standards Setting Subcommittee of the Institute of Electrical and Electronics Engineers (IEEE). In 1999, the federal Radio Frequency Interagency Work Group (RFIAWG) identified fourteen flaws in the IEEE standards. These include that the standards:

- were not based on any studies of RF field exposure to humans.
- were not based on any studies of exposure to modulated RF emissions.

- did not consider whether or how bodily tissues—the brain, bone marrow, heart, skin, etc.—are affected differently by exposure to RF fields.
- did not consider chronic, repeated or long-term exposure to low-intensity RF radiation. They addressed only a six-minute (cell phone) exposure at high intensity.
- did not consider high-quality published studies about health impacts.
- excluded research on long-term, low-level exposures; neurological and behavioral effects; and micronuclei assay studies relevant to cancer.

Despite RFIAWG's letter, Congress, the FCC, the FDA and the IEEE have not addressed these flaws.

1999

The FDA nominated RF radiation as a research topic of the National Toxicology Program (NTP). The FDA stated, "It is not scientifically possible to guarantee that those non-thermal levels of microwave radiation, which do not cause deleterious effects for relatively short exposure, will not cause long-term adverse health effects."

Fifteen years later, in 2014, the NTP study is "in progress." It only addresses exposure to cell phones—not to cellular antennas, Wi-Fi, or "smart" meters.

2001

In *Report 01-545* (gao.gov/new.items/d01545.pdf), the Government Accounting Office (GAO) criticized the FCC statement, "Cell Phones Cause Medical Problems is Fiction." The GAO report concluded that "it will likely be many more years before a definitive conclusion can be reached on whether mobile phone emissions pose any risk to human health." Responding to the GAO's criticism, the FCC's Office of Engineering and

Technology agreed that their "characterization could be misleading, because it implies that the health issue is settled."

2003

RFIAWG identified three more flaws in the IEEE's proposed changes to its cell phone safety standard. The IEEE proposal:

- classified the pinna of the ear as an extremity, the same as feet, ankles and hands, allowing the outer ear more radiation exposure.
- relaxed RF field exposure standards without giving rationale for doing so.
- ignored differences in exposed tissue types, without explanation.

RFIAWG received no response about these points.

2005

NTP stated why the FDA-nominated RF radiation human exposure study is necessary: "Current data are insufficient to draw definitive conclusions concerning the adequacy of these guidelines to be protective against any non-thermal effects of chronic exposures. Most scientific organizations that have reviewed the results from laboratory studies conducted to-date, however, have concluded that they are not sufficient to estimate potential human health cancer risks from low-level RFR exposures and long-term, multi-dose animal studies are needed."

2007–2008

At the request of the FDA and the Cellular Telephone and Internet Association (CTIA), the National Academies of Science (NAS) held a workshop to identify research needs on RF radiation exposure in preparation for publishing a report on its findings. The NAS Report stated that the research basis of the FCC's RF radiation safety policy does not consider a number of factors needed to protect the public's health (nap.edu/catalog.php?record_id=12036), including:

- differences in short-term v. long-term exposure.
- exposure to pulsed RF radiation.
- multilateral exposures.
- multiple frequency exposures.
- non-thermal effects.
- differences in risk to children, pregnant women, the elderly, the infirmand people with medical implants.
- whether RF radiation exposure alters the biological effects of other chemical or physical agents.

Both RFIAWG and the NAS panel findings delineated deficiencies in the FCC's RF exposure regulations research record. The record is inadequate to establish credible safety policy for today's environment, where everyone is ubiquitously exposed to radiation.

2009

At the FDA's request, *BioInitiative Report* coeditors Cindy Sage, M.A. and David O. Carpenter, MD, MPH provided a private briefing about the non-thermal effects of RF radiation.

In response, the FDA has taken no action to evaluate or address the BioInitiative Report's *studies and analysis.*

2012

The GAO issued *Report GAO-12-771, Telecommunications: Exposure and Testing Requirements for Mobile Phones Should Be Reassessed.* It stated, "FCC should formally reassess and, if appropriate, change its current RF energy exposure limit and mobile phone testing requirements related to likely usage configurations, particularly when phones are held against the body. FCC noted that a draft document currently under consideration by FCC has the potential to address GAO's recommendations."

2013

While the government's job is to protect the public, regardless of the burden to industry, the FCC 13-39 First Report and Order, issued in March 2013, stated that the Commission intends to "adequately protect the public without imposing an undue burden on industry."

On June 4, the FCC posted to the Federal Register a *Notice of Inquiry (NOI)* "to determine whether there is a need for reassessment of the Commission radio frequency (RF) exposure limits and policies. The NOI acknowledges the research that has occurred in recent years and the changing nature of RF devices and their uses, and focuses on the propriety of the Commission's existing standards and policies, including its fundamental exposure guidelines and aspects of its equipment authorization process and policies as they relate to RF exposure in light of these changes since its rules were adopted."

&

Janet Newton, President of EMRPI: *Indeed, it is high time for the FCC to reassess its RF exposure limits and policies and "acknowledge the research that has occurred in recent years and the changing nature of RF devices and their uses." The research underlying current FCC RF policies was published before 1987. Statements from NAS, RFIAWG, FDA and NTP clearly show that to date, the question of adverse health effects from long-term exposure to low-intensity RF radiation to all subgroups of the American public has not been answered in the research record that underlies the FCC's RF field safety regulations. Its guidelines are based on incomplete research.*

When industry representatives say, "We follow FCC standards," they bend the truth, because the FCC operates by guidelines, which are not as certain as standards. (Standards are based on research of exposure to humans; guidelines are based on non-human studies.) When they say, "You have nothing to worry about," we can ask them about the scientific basis of their guidelines (see epidemiologist Dr. De-Kun Li's clear explanation of the flaws in FCC standards in the appendices).

LEGAL POSSIBILITIES THAT RESPECT PUBLIC HEALTH AND OUR ECOSYSTEM

An Amendment to Section 704 of the Telecommunications Act

Whitney North Seymour, Jr., who served as the U.S. Attorney for New York, was a New York State Senator, and cofounded the Natural Resource Defense Council, drafted an amendment to the Telecommunications Act, Section 704 (presented in chapter 2). Mr. Seymour's amendment states: "Section 704 (47 U.S.C. s 332[c] [7] [B] [iv]) is hereby amended as follows: Nothing contained herein shall prevent a state or local government or instrumentality thereof from adopting a reasonable precautionary setback policy regulating the placement of such facilities in close proximity to schools, playgrounds, daycare facilities, residential communities, health care facilities or similar areas or facilities."

Mr. Seymour's amendment would restore local governments' ability to make zoning decisions that protect their citizens' general welfare around telecom equipment. No new costs would be incurred with this amendment, nor would the industry be subject to lawsuits from equipment previously placed. The EMR Policy Institute seeks cosponsors for the amendment.

The Cell Phone Right-to-Know Act

Congress could also pass legislation that would require informed labeling for mobile devices. In 2012, then-Representative Dennis Kucinich introduced the Cell Phone Right to Know Act (HR 6358), which would require that the EPA (not the FCC) set safety standards for mobile devices; that the EPA base these standards on biological needs and revise them every two years. Kucinich's bill also provided funding for research on the health and environmental effects of radiation from wireless devices. In December 2012, the American Academy of Pediatrics (AAP) endorsed the Cell Phone Right to Know Act (see the AAP endorsement in the appendix).

While Congress did not pass the Cell Phone Right to Know Act in 2012, current representatives can reintroduce it. (Phone your Congresspeople and urge them to sponsor and support 2012 HR6358.)

Expand the Definition of Harmful Interference

In June 2013, when the FCC announced their new emission standards (which increase a mobile device's allowable specific absorption rate—SAR—by reclassifying the outer ear as an extremity), it also acknowledged that its definition of "harmful interference" applies only to communications broadcasts, and does not include *biological* harm.[6] Indeed, our regulations need to include health.

In response to the FCC 2013 Notice of Inquiry, the EMR Policy Institute proposed the following definition for biological harm: *Harmful interference includes acute, chronic or prolonged exposure to EMFs or RFs that endangers, degrades, obstructs or repeatedly interrupts biological functioning of a*

6 See www.commlawblog.com/2009/01/articles/broadcast/finding-the-harm-in-harmful-interference/; posted by Mitchell Lazarus.

person, plant, animal or ecosystem and results in adverse health effects or malfunctioning of a medical device.

See EMRPI's full definition of biological harmful interference in the Solutions chapter. To see the full EMRPI Comment to the FCC, go to EMRPolicy.org.

❦

Janet Newton, President of EMRPI: *Many people wonder how society would function if regulatory agencies recognized the biological effects of radiofrequencies, and we drastically reduced our use of mobile devices and services. I expect we would function like people did before wireless devices. We would relearn sitting down at cabled connections to make phone calls and send emails. We would return to richer human interaction.*

When Plessy v. Ferguson was overturned, in 1954, in Brown v. Board of Education, no one knew how we would survive without "separate but equal" bathrooms and schools for differently-colored people. Well, we did survive. We did evolve. And now it's time to revise telecommunications laws that do not serve the public health or our ecosystem.

9

Slingshots at Goliath

Just because a problem is difficult to solve is not a reason to deny that a problem exists. Solutions to difficult issues usually can't be expected until the issues are known and creative thinking is brought to bear. Implementing the safety standards proposed in the BioInitiative Report could be very expensive and also could disrupt life and economy as we know them if implemented abruptly and without careful planning. Action must balance risk to cost and benefit. However, "deny and deploy" strategies by industry should not be rewarded.

David Carpenter, MD, and Cindy Sage, MA, "Key Scientific Evidence and Public Health Policy Recommendations," *The BioInitiative 2007 Report*

I wonder: *When have people noticed that their behavior was destructive—and then changed their behavior?* Hundreds of years ago, Native American farmers found their soil depleted when they planted the same crop in the same soil year after year. They began to rotate planting beans, corn and squash, and nutrients in the soil—and vegetables—were replenished.

Around 1900, in New York City, orphaned babies were fed well and kept warm in orphanages. But many of them died. When caregivers realized that babies also need to be held and lovingly touched, the babies thrived.

During the 1930s, people whose lives had become unmanageable because of alcoholism began meeting to share their experience while they got sober. They wrote the Twelve-Step Program and formed Alcoholics Anonymous.

In 1989, after the Soviet Union broke up, Cuba lost its oil supply. Suddenly, gas wasn't even available for trucks that transported food. The government bought three million bikes and turned available land into small farms. Scientists developed bio-dynamic fertilizers and pesticides that were not petroleum-based. Communities got strengthened by neighborhood farmers' markets, public transportation, and shared TVs.

When toxic waste from factories and petroleum-based farms made key waterways undrinkable, some people developed *mycorestoration*, cultivation of mushrooms that eat sludge. The water became drinkable again.

When apartheid ended in South Africa, the country's new leaders established the Truth and Reconciliation Commission, which granted amnesty to perpetrators (including killers and torturers) who told the truth about their crimes and apologized directly to people who suffered. They also included several verses from the old national anthem in the new one.

Here is a partial list of actions taken by international government agencies and professional organizations in response to concerns about the health and environmental effects of exposure to radio frequency radiation:

In official comments to the FCC about guidelines for evaluation of electromagnetic effects of RF radiation (FCC Docket ET 93–62, November 9, 1993), *The Environmental Protection Agency* found that the FCC's exposure standards are "seriously flawed" (emrpolicy.org).

The Food and Drug Administration commented to the FCC on November 10, 1993, that "FCC rules do not address the issue of long-term, chronic exposure to radio frequency fields" (emrpolicy.org Exhibit 46).

In 1999, the *Radio frequency Interagency Work Group* wrote a letter to IEEE SCC28, in which they identified fourteen issues that "need to be addressed to provide a strong and credible rationale to support RF exposure guidelines" (tinyurl.com/btfpae2).

In 1994, in comments to the FCC, the *Amateur Radio Relay League's Bio-Effects Committee* (ARRL) wrote that "The FCC's standard does not protect against non-thermal effects."

In 2003, the *American Bird Conservancy and Forest Conservation Council* sued the FCC because millions of migratory birds were disoriented by microwave radiation emitted by cell towers—and they were crashing into the towers (ewire.com/display.cfm/Wire_ID/1498).

In 2004, the *International Association of Fire Fighters* declared that it opposes communication antennas on fire stations (emrpolicy.org; iaff.org/HSFacts/CellTowerFinal.asp).

In 2007, *The European Environmental Agency*, Europe's top environmental watchdog, called for immediate action to reduce exposure to radiation from Wi-Fi, mobile phones, and their masts (eea.europa.eu/highlights/radiation-risk-from-everyday-devices:assessed).

In 2008, *public libraries in Paris, France* removed Wi-Fi from their buildings because of librarians' health concerns (accessmylibrary.com/coms2/summary_0286-35451555_ITM).

In 2008, the *Progressive Librarians Guild* recommended against wireless technology in libraries (libr.org/plg/wifiresolution.php).

In 2008, the *National Academy of Sciences* issued a report, "Identification of Research Needs Relating to Adverse Health Effects of Wireless Communication" (nap.edu/catalog.php?record_id=12036).

In 2008, *The International Commission on Electromagnetic Safety* (comprised of scientists from 16 nations) recommended limiting cell phone use by children, teenagers, pregnant women, and the elderly (icems.eu/resolution.htm).

In 2008, the *Russian National Committee for Non-Ionizing Radiation Protection* warned that cell phones are unsafe even for short conversations. Children under 16, pregnant women, epileptics, and people with memory loss, sleep disorders, and neurological diseases should never use cell phones (radiationresearch.org/pdfs/mcnirp_children.pdf).

In 2008, the *University of Pittsburg's Cancer Institute* warned that children should never use a cell phone except in an emergency (post-gazette.com/pg/08205/898803-114.stm).

In November 2009, an international team of physicians and scientists met in Seletun, Norway and created the *Seletun Scientific Statement* to urge new, biologically-based public exposure standards to protect public health worldwide regarding electromagnetic fields and radio frequency radiation (A. Fragopoulou et al, "Scientific panel on electromagnetic field health risks: Consensus points, recommendations, and rationales," *Reviews on Environmental Health*, vol. 25, no. 4 (2010): 307–317.).

In 2009, more than 50 scientists from 16 countries signed *The Porto Alegre Resolution*, an urgent call for more research based on "the body of evidence that indicates that exposure to electromagnetic fields interferes with basic human biology."

The U.S. Fish and Wildlife Service urged Congress to investigate the potential relationship between wireless devices and bee colony collapse in May, 2009 (see electromagnetichealth.org/electromagnetichealth-blog/emf-and-warnke-report-on-bees-birds-and-mankind/).

The government of *Frankfurt, Germany,* stated that it will not install Wi-Fi in its schools until it is proven harmless (see magdahavas.com/wordpress/wp-content/uploads/2010/09/German_Swiss_Wifi_In-Schools_Warn.pdf, p.5.).

In 2010, *France* prohibited pre-K through high school students' use of a mobile phone during school. France Environmental Law, Article 183.

In 2010, *municipalities in California, Hawaii, Maine, and Maryland* passed resolutions creating moratoriums on "smart" meters (for updates, check emfsafetynetwork.org or stopsmartmeters.org).

The World Health Organization classified radio frequency electromagnetic fields as a possible carcinogen on May 31, 2011. Also that month, the *WHO* added multiple chemical sensitivity and electro-hypersensitivity (EHS) on its International Classification of Diseases.

In May 2011, the *Parliamentary Assembly Council of Europe (PACE)* released a resolution, "Potential Dangers of Electromagnetic Fields and Their Effect on the Environment." It states "for children in general, and particularly in schools and classrooms, give preference to wired Internet connections, and strictly regulate the use of mobile phones by schoolchildren on school premises (assembly.coe.int/Mainf.asp?link=Documents/AdoptedText.tal.ERES1815.htm).

In January 2012, *The American Academy of Environmental Medicine* called for an immediate moratorium on "smart" meters until "serious health issues" related to their installation are resolved (see the appendix).

In January 2012, the *Santa Cruz, California Board of Supervisors* voted to continue a temporary moratorium on "smart" meter installations in the county, accepting the Public Health Department's report that "smart" meters harm health.

The Ontario English Catholic Teachers' Association (OECTA) expressed concern in February 2012 about Wi-Fi in the workplace (magdahavas.com/ontario-english-catholic-teachers-association-wi-fi-in-the-workplace).

In March 2012, *four Vermont communities rejected "smart" meters: Bennington, Dorset, Manchester, and Sandgate* (www.wakeupoptout.org).

The Austrian Medical Association created guidelines for the diagnosis and treatment of EMF-related health problems and illnesses in March, 2012 (aerztekammer.at/documents/10618/976981/EMF-Guideline.pdf).

In June 2012, *Women's College Hospital* in Toronto stated that family doctors must learn to detect symptoms of exposure to radiation from wireless devices—including disrupted sleep, headaches, nausea, dizziness, heart palpitations, memory problems, and rashes (womenscollegehospital.ca/news-and-events/connect/the-effects-of-invisible-waves).

Following a report from *a committee formed by India's Ministry of Communications and Information Technology*, India decided, in July 2012, to reduce its limit on radiation emitted by antennas *tenfold*. Currently, India's radiation exposure limit for antennas is 9.2 w/m2 (watts per square meter). Russia's limit is 0.2 w/m2. China's is 0.4 w/m2. In the U.S., Canada and Japan, the exposure limit is 12 w/m2. With the new ruling, India will lower its standard to 0.92 w/m2. Telecom operators claim that reducing antenna power means that mobile devices will have to work harder and thereby, they will increase users' exposure. To provide sufficient coverage, the companies claim that they'll need to install more antennas (articles.economictimes.indiatimes.com/2012-07-18/news/32730933_1_radiation-exposure-mobile-towers-emf).

In July 2012, *The Maine Supreme Judicial Court* ruled that the state's Public Utilities Commission had not adequately addressed safety concerns about "smart" meters installed by Central Maine Power Company. Maine regulators will now investigate the meters' health and safety issues.

In August 2012, *Israel's Ministry of Health* called for a ban on Wi-Fi in schools (norad4u.blogspot.co.il/2012/08/this-is-translation-to-english-of.html).

In November 2012, the *High Court of Rajasthan*, India's largest state geographically, ordered all cell towers removed from the vicinity of schools, colleges, hospitals and playgrounds because radiation is "hazardous to life."

On July 5, 2013, *India's Supreme Court* upheld this decision.

In December 2012, *the American Academy of Pediatrics* endorsed the Cell Phone Right to Know Act because of its "emphasis on examining the effects of radio frequency (RF) energy on vulnerable populations, including children and pregnant women." See the appendix.

In February 2013, the *Administrative Appeals Tribunal of the Australian Federal Court* legally recognized the health effects of electromagnetic radiation in a workplace compensation case. Because his employer required his trial use of electronic equipment, Dr. Alexander McDonald's health suffered (austiii.edu/au/au/cases/cth/aat/2013/105.html).

In February 2013, *Belgium's Public Health Minister* announced that sales of mobile phones to children under seven will be prohibited, as will advertisements for mobile phones during children's TV, radio, and Internet programming (expatica.com/be/news/belgian-news/TMag-Mobile-phones-to-be-banned-for-children_259994.html).

In a February 8, 2013, letter to the Los Angeles Unified School District, *Martha Herbert, MD, PhD, a pediatric neurologist at Harvard Medical School*, wrote, "EMF/RFR from Wi-Fi and cell towers can exert a disorganizing effect on the ability to learn and remember, and can also be destabilizing to immune and metabolic function. This will make it harder for some children to learn, particularly those who are already having problems.... I urge you to step back from your intention to go with Wi-Fi in the LAUSD, and instead opt for wired technologies.... It will be easier for you to make a healthier decision now than to undo a misguided decision later."

In March 2013, the Los Angeles Teacher's Union passed a resolution to ensure safety from hazardous electromagnetic fields in schools, including from wireless technologies (nea.org/assets/docs/nea-resolutions-2012-13.pdf).

In March 2013, *Australia's Radiation Protection and Nuclear Safety Agency* advised parents to limit children's use of mobile and cordless phones and to keep monitors at least a meter away from babies' beds in order to minimize their exposure to EMR (perthnow.com.au/lifestyle/technology/parents-urged-to-limit-childrens-use-of-mobiles-cordless-phone-under-new-health-warnings/story-fn7bsi10-1226589473040).

In June 2013, British Airways announced in the *Daily Telegraph* that its new aircraft will not have Wi-Fi.

In August 2013, the *Elementary Teachers Federation of Ontario*, representing 76,000 teachers, recommended to all school boards that cell phones be turned off in classrooms to protect students' and teachers' health. It also voted that all Wi-Fi transmitters be clearly visible and labeled as part of a hazard control program (c4st.ca).

Cole County, Missouri Judge Patricia Joyce put an indefinite hold, in August 2013, on the Uniform Wireless Communications Infrastructure Deployment Act. This state act exempts cell towers from virtually all local zoning regulations. Six cities claimed that the law violated the Missouri constitution. Judge Joyce agreed, ruling, "The implementation, enforcement, application or assertion of any provision of HB 331 or HB 345 will subject the plaintiffs to the unwarranted burdens of unconstitutional laws and immediate and irreparable injury, loss or damage will result in the absence of relief and preservation of the status quo." Matt Kalish, "Cole County Judge Shoots Down Attempt to Limit Cell Phone Tower Fees," *Eldorado Springs Sun*, 9.5.13.

In August 2013, *Mumbai, India*'s most populated city, voted to prohibit antennas 1)in the vicinity of schools, colleges, orphanages, child rehabilitation centers and nursing homes; and 2)from being directed toward such buildings. The city also voted to prohibit installation of antennas on residential rooftops without the consent of every person on the top floor as well as 70% of residents below the top floor. The city intends to dismantle 3,200 illegal rooftop antennas (prd34.blogspot.com/2013/08/reminder-comments-to-fcc-due-this.html).

10

Living with Ourselves and Others in this Virtual Season

It will be humbling to work with you.

Said by a tutor to her student on learning that the student would need Wi-Fi and a wireless printer dismantled during his lessons

In 1963, after *Silent Spring* introduced the hazards of pesticides to the American public, Rachel Carson testified before Congress. "I hope this committee will give serious consideration to a much-neglected problem: that of the right of the citizen to be secure in his own home against the intrusion of poisons applied by other persons.... This is or should be one of the basic human rights." Carson's testimony led to Congress creating the Environmental Protection Agency.

Half a century later, our relationship to modern technologies remains complex. Utility companies have installed "smart" meters without testing their biological effects or requesting our informed consent. Telecom companies have installed antennas, 4G and WiMax throughout cities and towns, again without testing or informed consent about their biological effects. Workplaces, schools, and neighbors have installed Wi-Fi with the assumption that it is safe; churches and schools have installed antennas in order to receive rent from telecom companies—also with the assumption that such transmitters do not harm. And nearly everyone subscribes to mobile services or has family members who do.

Most peoples' jobs require them to have mobile service. Students who do not have Internet access would be considered handicapped. How do we cope with the fact that almost everyone alive now is at least partly responsible for the radiation that "intrudes" our homes? Facing this riddle may not result in viable solutions. Ignoring the riddle does not make it go away.

In 1997, I bought a computer. I used it for twenty minutes, then suddenly felt twitching at the back of my neck. The symptoms morphed into the flu. Over the next few days, I used the computer for brief stints. Each time, I saw flickering on the screen that seemed to disturb my nervous system. Within the week, I returned the computer.

I'm a writer. I *really* wanted a word processor and Internet access. Over the next several years, I tried screen shields, LCD screens, projector monitors, behavioral optometry and special glasses. I bought and returned a dozen computers. Nothing helped.

I considered the situation my personal problem. I hired helpers who read my email to me and typed my dictated replies. I met a woman whose computer can still take the four-inch discs from my old word processor and translate them into modern Word. So, I can still publish.

Then, in 2008, one of four gold crowns I'd had installed in 1997 (a few months before I bought the first computer that made me so sick) fell off. I asked another dentist to re-glue the loose one. "You know," the new dentist told me, "there's mercury here."

"No," I assured him. "I had all my mercury removed in 1992."

The new dentist handed me a mirror, and I saw silver amalgam on my uncrowned tooth. Alas. Mixing metals in a moist environment creates oral galvanism, an electric current that runs through my body.

Call dental work the likely source of my flicker sensitivity. (FYI, I believe the dentist gave me fresh mercury under gold crowns because he thought that these were the most enduring materials that he had. In the U.S., installing such materials is still perfectly legal.)

By 2010, I had all of the gold and mercury removed from my teeth. A hair test in 2013 revealed I've still got extremely high levels of mercury, which my doctor attributes to dental work and consuming fish.

I'm still "flicker-sensitive." I experience tingling, tremors, and ear ringing 24/7. My eyes are often blurred; to read, I need at least a 14 point font. My heart rate can change just from being near a Wi-Fi hot spot. Being in a place with fluorescent lights can shift me into high alert. At night, I often feel like a radio station that primarily plays *static*.

Does exposure to electrosmog exacerbate my symptoms? I know of no place that "tests" how I respond to an environment without magnetic and/or radio-frequency fields.

Numerous studies find that at least three percent of the population experiences radio-wave sickness.[1] Yet other studies report that when toxic agents (like mercury) are combined with exposure to magnetic fields, damage is enhanced.[2]

---

1 P. Levallois et al, "Study of self-reported hypersensitivity to electromagnetic fields in California," *Environmental Health Perspectives,* vol. 110, suppl 4 (2002): 619–23; L. Hillert et al, "Prevalence of self-reported hypersensitivity to electric or magnetic fields in a population-based questionnaire survey," *Scandinavian Journal of Work, Environment, and Health,* vol. 28, no. 1 (2002): 33–41; N. Schreier et al, "The Prevalence of symptoms attributed to electromagnetic field exposure: A cross-sectional representative survey in Switzerland," *Soz Praventivmed,* vol. 51, no. 4 (2006): 202–9.

2 J. Juutilainen et al, , "Do extremely low frequency magnetic fields enhance the effects of environmental carcinogens? A meta-analysis

Relating respectfully with other people (who mostly want wider, faster coverage for their devices and do not perceive that mobile phones, Wi-Fi, fluorescent lights, or transmitters affect health) leaves me challenged.

Once, visiting friends, I was seated across from a clock that flashed red numbers into the air, like a hologram. My partner, Brooke, saw my distress. "Katie," he said calmly, "let's switch seats."

After we moved, the clock *f+l!i*c?k#e*r!!e=d! in my peripheral view. The stimulation felt like an attack. "If you don't unplug that thing immediately," I told our hosts, "I'm going to get violent."

My host unplugged the clock. I phoned the next day to apologize and explain flicker sensitivity. My friends said, "Don't worry about it." But that was the end of our friendship.

Apparently, many people struggle to navigate our digitalized world. Here are some of their stories.

⚭

Jacqueline Holly, 53, Wisconsin: *Since 4G and three (electric, gas and water) wireless meters arrived in my town, I cannot sleep in my house. I might sleep an hour, but my joints get so stiff and achy that by morning, I can barely walk. My thinking gets dull. I cannot tolerate dulled thinking.*

Since March 2011, I leave my house every night at 10:30 with a cross from my childhood on my car's dashboard, and sleep in a shopping center parking lot.

I tried sleeping at a park, but a security guard there knocked on my window and woke me. That was scary. He figured I was having family problems, and said I couldn't stay. I tried another shopping center, but its power lines caused so much

of experimental studies," *International Journal of Radiation Biology*, vol. 82, no. 1(2006): 1–12.

pressure in my head and chest that I couldn't sleep. From the lot where I am now, I can see a cell tower about a quarter of a mile away. On cold nights, I wear three layers of hunters' socks, long underwear, two sweatpants and sweatshirts. I slip into a sleeping bag, then cover myself with two aluminized plastic blankets, which seem to shield me from the cell tower's emissions. On a good night, I sleep for six hours. I wake with tingling (and condensation dripping onto the sleeping bag), but my thinking is still clear. Usually, I return home to my husband and younger son by seven a.m.

My husband tried to make a Faraday cage with metal screens to block radiation from reaching our bed. Perhaps because he didn't seal the bottom properly, it didn't work. We're just not technicians. Shielding canopies are expensive, and interaction between highly conductive shielding material and the electric fields from wiring in the walls can actually make the situation worse.

My doctor recognizes chemical sensitivities, but he doesn't believe that "smart" meters could cause problems. He is open to literature, so I've begun to offer him some from physicians' organizations.

I have two masters degrees, a marriage of twenty-two years and two nearly grown children. People say I look good. They don't see the numbness and tingling I experience all the time, which gets stronger when I'm in a building with "smart" meters or Wi-Fi. They don't see the head pain that comes when someone uses a cell phone near me.

ꕥ

Claire Pollack, 42, New York: *One evening, after learning that the FCC had proposed eliminating landlines, I sat on our sofa, paralyzed. Suddenly, my husband started ranting: "I hate you! I wish I'd never met you! I wish you'd never been born!" Somehow,*

I knew he was just venting frustration and helplessness. I told him, "I believe you. I see that you think these things right now."

"I do!*" he insisted.*

"I get it," I said sincerely.

And then his rage dissipated. It was over.

Jason can't change laws that value technology more than nature. He can't convince our neighbors to quit their Wi-Fi and get cabled Internet access. He can't find us a radio-free zone. "Really," he said, "I hate myself, because nothing I do helps.*"*

As I see it, lots of people have "insane" outbursts these days. They might be related to the proliferation of radiation from wireless devices; they might not. But every "sensitive" person I know has a spouse or children who use mobile phones and Wi-Fi and GPS devices and baby monitors, and friends who think that fluorescent lights are good for our ecosystem. Everyone has a neighbor who thinks we're just intent on spreading "fearful" information.

To survive, my peacemaking skills need constant honing.

⌘

Anne O'Connor, 62, Massachusetts: *Since he was conceived, my grandson has been exposed to two smartphones, several "smart" meters, Wi-Fi and a GPS device. My younger daughter attends a prestigious college that has proudly eliminated all of its landlines. How do I discuss my concerns with my children without creating agitation?*

⌘

Ginger Farver (chapter 1 story): *After my son died and I learned about the harm caused by wireless devices, I got very angry. Angry that San Diego State and other schools do not take responsibility, inform their students and staff about radiation emitted by wireless devices or install protective policies. I had rage for the telecom corporations, the government and* *individual subscribers who endanger themselves and everyone who lives or works near an antenna.*

To give my anger a place, I've distributed flyers about the dangers of non-ionizing radiation. At town council meetings, I've warned my neighbors about the harm caused by "smart" meters.

I realize that the broader situation is far beyond human control now. But we still need to start with ourselves. Since each person's use of a wireless device forces radiation exposure on others, each person who decreases their use reduces everyone's exposure.

To educate and support each other while we face these inconvenient truths, parents and young people need to get together.

As often as I can remember, I say thanks to life itself, to that Power that is greater than all the utility and telecom companies combined.

11
Solutions

While running Microsoft's sales and marketing departments for businesses in Canada and the Central U.S., I saw technology's positive impact on peoples' lives. I still see that. But until now, many of us have missed the boat about technology's harmful effects. We need to recognize the scientific evidence that radiation emitted by electronics and wireless devices can and does lead to autism, Alzheimer's, cancer, memory issues, inability to think clearly and much more. Pregnant women and children are especially vulnerable. We need to recognize Electro-hypersensitivity, and to protect people who want to avoid involuntary exposure to radio-frequency radiation with radio-free zones. My organization supports informing the public about technology's biological effects and revising safety standards on electronics and wireless devices so that our biological limitations are respected. We are not Canadians for No Technology. We are Canadians for Safe Technology.

—Frank Clegg, former President, Microsoft Canada and founding CEO of c4st.org

First Steps

With this book, I have aimed to encourage dialogue about the benefits of our rapidly expanding electronic revolution—and the unintended and mostly unrecognized problems that it causes to our health and environment. The following solutions are culled from international sources. They can move us toward a safer electrical grid, safer electronics, safer telecommunications—and a healthier world.

First Steps for Individuals and Society

1. Recognize that electricity, electronics, and wireless devices have brought great benefits to humanity. Recognize that electricity and electromagnetic radiation can harm health and the environment (*BioInitiative Report 2012;* The Seletun Scientific Statement 2009; and EMR Policy Institute—see EMR Policy's proposed definition of biological harmful interference on page 188).
2. Recognize that electronic innovations and inventions have outpaced testing, monitoring, and regulating health effects. Recognize that safety standards do not exist for children, pregnant women, people with medical implants, or other vulnerable populations. Recognize that current standards do not consider the effects of exposure to second-hand radiation, multiple frequencies, or multiple transmitters (FCC Notice of Inquiry 13–39).
3. Commit to guiding ourselves by the Precautionary Principle and first do no harm. Do not deploy or purchase any new technology until third party, independent testing proves that it does not cause biological harm (see "Precautionary Principle" defined in the glossary).

Next Steps

Next Steps for Legislators

1. Mandate a clearly stated federal law that FCC standards do not preempt the ability of injured citizens to go to court and recover damages caused by the trespass of electromagnetic radiation into their bodies (EMRpolicy.org).
2. Mandate Whitney North Seymour Jr.'s amendment to Section 704 of the Telecommunications Act, which will allow localities to determine their own setback policy on telecom equipment (EMRpolicy.org).
3. In Congress, reintroduce and mandate the Cell Phone Right to Know Act (HR 6358 2012). It will require telecom companies to allow epidemiologists to access records of cell phone users for health research, give the EPA authority to determine biological safety standards on cell phones and require SAR labeling on mobile phones. All EMR-emitting devices should be included in this Act (12.12.12 letter from the American Academy of Pediatrics, in the appendix).
4. Mandate third-party testing of SARs and warning labels on all electronic devices that 1)show a picture of how far radiation penetrates the head when the device is near it and 2) state, "This device emits electromagnetic radiation, exposure to which may cause brain cancer. Users, especially children and pregnant women, should keep this device away from the head and body" (Maine Children's Wireless Protection Act, proposed by legislator Andrea Boland; American Academy of Pediatrics; electromagnetichealth.org).
5. Enforce National Environmental Policy Act (NEPA) requirements of Environmental Assessment before deploying new technology near schools or sensitive habitats (epa.gov).
6. Repeal the FCC's reclassifying the pinna (outer part) of the ear as an extremity in its 2013 Reassessment of RF Exposure Limits and Policies (Radio Frequency Interagency Work Group, 2003 letter to FCC).
7. Allow people with medical implants and Electro-hypersensitivity reasonable accommodation (i.e., shut off wireless devices and services, metal detectors, inventory control, and

RFID systems) in public spaces (1991 Americans with Disabilities Act).

8. To provide immediate relief, allow every ratepayer in every state the option of a mechanical, analog meter for their utilities.

Next Steps for Regulators

1. Mandate a nationwide, standardized, and regulated electrical code—instead of our current (voluntary) National Fire Protection Association-National Electrical Code. Recognize that "interference" can harm electrical equipment *and* cause thermal and non-thermal effects that harm human health and the environment. OSHA should regulate this code for workers' safety; FDA should regulate the electrical grid's impact on public health, including medical devices and equipment; and EPA should regulate the grid's environmental impacts. This code should be applied to the "smart" grid and "smart" appliances and all sources of electricity, including unconventional sources (BioIniative.org; HR 6358 2012).
2. Revise our National Electrical Safety Code (NESC) so that there is no more than 1.0 mG (0.1 microtesla) of magnetic field within habitable space (BioInitiative 2012, p. 37).
3. NESC must also require utilities to separate neutrals and grounds correctly to prevent return current from flowing over the earth, metallic water and gas piping, building steel, and other conductive materials—and to prevent shocking or even electrocuting people in showers or swimming pools (Donald Zipse, "Are the National Electrical Code and the National Electrical Safety Code Hazardous to Your Health?" *Industrial Commercial Power Systems Technical Conference*, 1999).
4. Mandate single-point grounding-transformer isolation on all transformers so that neutral wires are not shared, and ground current and magnetic fields are significantly reduced (*Practical Grounding, Bonding, Shielding and Surge Protection*, by G. Vijayaraghavan, M. Brown and M. Barnes, Newnes/Elsevier, 2004, p. 237).

5. Quantify levels of electromagnetic radiation that cause biological harm. Establish a standard for reaching safe levels for all segments of the population and the environment (BioInitiative.org; note: in 1971, OSHA issued a protection guide for workers' exposure to RF radiation [29 CFR 1910.97]. This guide was later ruled to be advisory, not mandatory. osha.gov/SLTC/radio frequencyradiation/).
6. Mandate regulations that limit electrical and electromagnetic radiation to levels that protect human health and the environment (BioInitiative.org; HR 6358 2012).
7. Require periodic testing (by independent third parties) for the presence of hazardous levels, similar to current testing for and enforcement of air quality standards. Require mitigation when hazardous levels are reached, followed by retesting (EMRpolicy.org).
8. The FCC should require installation of sensors at all building-mounted and tower-mounted transmitter locations. Emissions levels should be recorded on a regular, ongoing basis and sent to a computer interface via a cabled phone or fiber optic line. These readings should be monitored and posted on a website accessible to the public. High levels should be mitigated promptly (EMRpolicy.org, Americans Beware).
9. The FCC should promote cabled Internet in residences, at public institutions and in localities. Fiber optics should be installed for *cabled* (not wireless) services, including Internet, TV, and telephone (EMRpolicy.org).
10. Congress should fund the FDA to regulate the effects of RF signals and emissions on people who depend on medical devices and medical equipment (Center for Devices and Radiological Health *and* Electronic Product Radiation Control Program at FDA).
11. Require licensed electricians to learn (through continuing education) to periodically identify and eliminate wiring errors on utility wiring and in public and private buildings that generate magnetic fields and ground current—and that may cause biological harm (*Soares Book on Grounding and*

Bonding, 10th ed. International Association of Electrical Inspectors, 2008, p. 429).

12. Require health care providers, educators, electricians, city planners, architects, electronics designers, solar and wind power manufacturers, and others to take annual continuing education about how electronics, wireless devices, and transmitters create hazards for children, pregnant women, people with medical implants, people with EHS, and the environment, similar to OSHA and EPA mandated periodic training to deal with hazardous materials (OSHA.gov, EPA.gov and, for example, 29 Code Federal Regulation).

Next Steps for Utility and Telecommunications Companies

1. Replace every digital wireless transmitting utility meter with an analog mechanical one (BioInitiative.org; see also letters from epidemiologist De-Kun Li, MD and the American Academy for Environmental Medicine in the appendix).
2. Keep TV and radio broadcast facilities far from populated areas. Do not allow them to be grand-fathered (EMRpolicy.org).
3. Maintain phone landlines, a known, safe technology (BioInitiative.org).

Next Steps for Manufacturers

1. Recognize that high frequencies generated by linear and switch-mode power supplies (SMPSs) generate square waves and harmonics that interfere with electronic equipment *and* may cause biological harm. Eliminate fluorescent lights, including compact fluorescent bulbs (CFLs), which use electronic ballasts (aka SMPSs); they generate high frequency harmonics, and they usually contain mercury. Replace them with bulbs such as LEDs that save energy and do not generate square waves and harmonics. Eliminate dimmer switches that generate square waves and harmonics; replace them with dimmers that do not generate harmonics or with standard switches. Revisit standards for electronics and appliances, including 12-volt DC electronics and appliances, that

are currently used on boats, RVs, and in some solar-powered homes (BioInitiative.org).

2. Design solar-powered systems that do not generate high frequency fields. Eliminate DC-AC inverters. Whenever possible, use propane or DC-powered appliances and electronics in solar-powered homes and buildings.
3. Create safer electric and hybrid cars, whose existing computerized systems (charging, LCD display, windows, etc.) trap drivers and passengers in a metal box filled with electromagnetic fields.
4. Create safer medical implants by installing a hazard-overload interrupter in every implant, similar to ground-fault interrupters in household wiring (Dr. Gary Olhoeft).
5. Reduce or eliminate ads for wireless devices that target children, as France has done. Reduce or eliminate depictions of substance abuse or violence in films or videos and create more pro-social programs (American Academy of Pediatrics; Kaiser Permanente).

Next Steps for Healthcare Providers

1. Require continuing education for physicians, first responders, public health assessors, and other health care providers about creating electrically safe living, learning, and working environments for pregnant women, children, people with medical implants, and those with Electro-hypersensitivity. Physicians must be trained to recognize Electro-hypersensitivity; to educate parents about creating an electrically safe environment for children; to perform common procedures (i.e., dental work and hernia surgery) safely on people with medical implants (Austrian Medical Association Guidelines, aerztekammer.at/documents/10618/976981/EMF-Guideline.pdf; Dr. Gary Olhoeft).
2. The AAP encourages pediatricians to ask, at every well-child visit, *How much recreational screen time does your child or teen consume daily? Is there a TV or Internet-connected device in the child's bedroom?* Physicians should encourage parents to establish a plan for all home media use (*Pediatrics* 2013;132958–961).

3. Create centers that treat children and adults who use mobile devices addictively, similar to centers that address gambling, alcohol, and drug addictions.
4. Require every hospital to employ an electrical interference specialist (as many already do) to monitor potentially hazardous interference between devices *and* between personnel, patients, and devices. Health care providers should educate themselves and their clients about plausible and known risks to health caused by RF fields; they should encourage precautionary behavior among themselves and their clients.

Next Steps for Schools (including Trade Schools) and Libraries

1. Remove Wi-Fi and wireless devices from schools and libraries. Provide wired learning environments for students and faculty (Dr. Martha Herbert and Cindy Sage, MA, "Autism and EMF? Plausibility of a pathophysiological link; parts 1 and 2," *Pathophysiology* 2013).
2. Remove digital wireless transmitting utility meters from schools and libraries. Replace them with analog mechanical meters.
3. Provide guidance for educators to recognize Electro-hypersensitivity in children and the addictive nature of using interactive electronic devices and the Internet—similar to guidance issued by the CDC for identifying children with food allergies, preventing exposures and managing reactions (cdc.gov/healthyyouth/foodallergies/). Strengthen students' communication skills in non-electronic, eye-to-eye contact (*Alone Together*, by Sherry Turkle; see also "Children, Adolescents and the Media," a 10.28.13 Policy Statement from the AAP).
4. Eliminate fluorescent lights. Use incandescent or CLED lights.
5. Before granting licenses, master electricians and plumbers should require apprentices to identify and clear magnetic fields in their own homes.
6. Create institutes that teach people how to measure ELFs, RF fields, and SARs; how to identify whether electricity is safely installed; whether the levels of electromagnetic fields in an

area are safe; how to mitigate unsafe levels (and how to identify when an environment cannot be mitigated without major infrastructure changes); and how to live with fewer electronics.

Next Steps for Environmental, Citizen, Religious, and Professional Groups

1. Encourage awareness about the biological effects of emissions from electronics and wireless services on pregnant women, children, people with medical implants, and others. Encourage schools, doctors' offices, libraries, places of worship, restaurants, other areas of public accommodation—and your own workplace—to dismantle wireless services, including digital wireless utility meters.
2. As an immediate step to accommodate electrosensitive members, congregations could dismantle wireless services and request that members leave wireless devices at home for weekly or monthly gatherings.
3. To support surveys for magnetic and RF fields, libraries, schools, businesses, and civic organizations could purchase magnometers and RF meters (about $700 each) to loan or rent.
4. Push a solution-based agenda with local and federal legislators and regulators that will make our society safer and healthier (BioInitiative.org).

ꕥ

George Tabor, 66, retired nuclear structural inspector for the Navy: *For more than two decades, my work included inspecting nuclear power plants on submarines for structural errors. The Navy obeyed NAVSEA guidelines, which limit the amount of radiation that workers can be exposed to by the quarter and by the year. Every day, my body was tested to ensure that I was not exposed to more radiation than NAVSEA allowed. Over the years, standards changed, and we workers were allowed less exposure. Before the Navy let me work, I signed that I understood that I would be exposed to ionizing radiation, and that it could harm my health. I retired in 1995.*

Around 2007, city-wide Wi-Fi got installed in my town. "Smart" meters arrived in 2010. After these installations, my diabetes symptoms got worse, and I developed heart arrhythmia, sleep apnea and nervous tension. In the summer of 2013, a new device was put on the utility pole near my house. I've heard that it connects Wi-Fi, the "smart" grid and emergency response communications. Is this true? *I don't know.* Is this safe? *I don't know. But when I stand on my porch, I feel dizzy, like someone kicked me in the knees. I get headaches and frequent nightmares. I lose my strength and become easily irritable.*

I removed all wireless devices and services from my house, but I still don't feel well here. Several times, I've slept on a friend's sofa a few towns away. I bought an oximeter, which measures the oxygen in my blood. According to my doctor, a reading of 97% or higher means I'm getting the oxygen I need. Seventeen miles out of town, I'm at a healthy, 99%. In town, I usually measure 88% to 95%. Once, it measured 83% in town.

I got an Acoustimeter from lessemfs.com to identify hot spots of extremely low frequencies and radiofrequencies around my house and the city. On my porch, I usually find electric fields of 0.07 to 1.0 volts per meter. Downtown, 3.0, 4.0 and even 5.0 volts per meter are common. These are not safe levels, especially for 24/7 exposure. They are likely Wi-Fi and cell phone signals, maybe also TV or taxi dispatch signals.

The BioInitiative 2012 Report *advises limiting electric field exposure to 0.03 volts per meter. The EPA advises keeping exposure to less than 0.13. The FCC says to keep it to less than 2.0 volts per meter.*

Clearly, it's high time for a government agency to determine, monitor and enforce safe levels of ELFs and RF fields—just like the Navy does for workers exposed to ionizing radiation.

⚮

David Carpenter, MD, Professor of Environmental Medicine at SUNY/Albany and coeditor of ***The BioInitiative Report*****, in a statement for the President's Cancer Panel; January 27, 2009:** The BioInitiative Report *presents recommendations for standards of EMF exposure that are based on the epidemiological evidence in human populations. For ELF (extremely low frequency) EMFs, the proposed standard is 1 mG (0.1 uT), to be compared with the current International Commission on Non-ionizing Radiation Protection (ICNRP) standard of 1,000 mG (100 uT). For RF radiation, the proposed standard is 0.1 μW/cm2, to be compared with the U.S. FCC standard of 583 μW/cm2 for 875 MHz cell phone frequency and 1,000 μW/cm2 in the frequency range of 1800 to 1950 MHz.*

The differences between these numbers show the magnitude of the problem. There is no question that a sudden imposition of standards so drastically different from those existing would impose hardship. There is also no question that human studies clearly indicate that existing standards do not protect human health.

The benefits to society derived from electricity and wireless communications are significant, and certainly none of us is willing to return to the pre-electric age. However, it is imperative that society at least acknowledge the disparities between current standards and current evidence of risk of cancer.

Rigid and sudden imposition of the standards we propose is unrealistic, but these levels are appropriate goals that could at least be approached by a combination of development of new technology and changes in behaviors.[1]

---

1 D. O. Carpenter, "Electromagnetic fields and cancer: The cost of doing nothing," *Reviews on Environmental Health*, vol. 25, no. 1, (2010): 75–80.

A Definition of Biological Harmful Interference Proposed by the EMR Policy Institute in its September 2013 Comment to the FCC:

Harmful interference includes acute, chronic or prolonged exposure to RF signals and emissions that endangers, degrades, obstructs, or repeatedly interrupts biological functioning of a person, plant, animal, or ecosystem, or that results in adverse health effects from malfunctioning of medical devices or equipment.

Biological harmful interference shall be defined as any negative change in a measurable biological, physiological or ecological parameter (outside the range within which it is regulated in normal circumstances with no exposure to the influence in question). *Examples of parameters that demonstrate biological effects caused by exposure to magnetic fields or RF fields include*:

- the EEG spindle frequency during sleep (reproducible within a person, not necessarily across a population);
- the brain metabolic rate based on brain scans of glucose metabolism;
- the rate of DNA breakage in healthy cells;
- disruption of the rate of calcium efflux through a cell's membrane;
- melatonin production and metabolism;
- insulin production and metabolism;
- heart rate and blood pressure variability;
- temperature (note that a temporary temperature change of 0.2° Fahrenheit shall be considered a biological effect, because a healthy body normally regulates temperature within a range smaller than this).

Examples of parameters that demonstrate harmful biological effects caused by magnetic and/or RF fields exposed to the environment include:

- the mortality rate of plants or animals;
- the incidence of deformed offspring of plants or animals;
- altered growth or morphology in plants or animals;
- behavioral changes (such as nesting, increased piping signaling of bees or altered feeding habits by any animal).

What Individuals Can Do

According to people who study remedies for exposure to environmental toxins, the first line of defense is to get away from the harmful element. This is especially true for pregnant women, babies, children, and the infirm. Since most of us live, work, and study in chronically exposed areas, decreasing exposure to EMR may be only minimally possible. But each of us can reduce our personal use of wireless devices.

Some studies show that people who do not have wireless devices (i.e., cell phones, cordless landlines, and Wi-Fi) in their homes do not activate stress hormones as much as those who do have such devices—including when both groups are exposed to RF fields from cell towers.[2] In other words, reducing your use of wireless devices may lower your stress levels, even when you are exposed to radiation from equipment beyond your control.

1. Make Sure Your Electrical System Is Properly Wired and That Your Home Does Not Have Magnetic Fields

Determine whether or not your home and workplace have EMFs. Use a portable AM radio as a gauss meter (the appendix has instructions) or rent a magnometer.

2 K. Buchner and H. Eger, "Changes of clinically important neurotransmitters under the influence of modulated RF fields: A long-term study under real-life conditions," *Umwelt-Medizin-Gesellschaft*, vol. 24, no. 1 (2011): 44–57.

Study Karl Riley's book, Tracing EMFs in Building Wiring and Grounding. *Find an electrician who's open to learning how to reduce magnetic fields within and around your home.* Note that the average house—whether old, new or remodeled—has several wiring errors. Many questions about exposure to magnetic fields and RFs are still unanswered, and few people (including electricians) know how to decrease EMFs.

If you identify power lines around your house that generate magnetic fields, work with your utility company to reduce them. Marv Loftness' book, *AC Powerline Interference Handbook*, provides an excellent guide.

If a light flickers even after you install a new bulb, hire an electrician to replace its switch and to check for a possible loose connection.

Avoid appliances with digital displays, since they generate magnetic fields. If your oven has a digital display, plug it into a power strip. Keep its digital display off, except when using the oven. Use a striker to light the burners.

Keep the trees near your power lines well-trimmed, since branches that contact power lines can create arcing. To avoid this problem if you're building a new house, plant bushes or small trees near the power lines.

Every few years, *hire an electrician to tighten the connections in your circuit breaker panel and in each outlet,* starting with the outlet nearest your breakers. A loose connection can create small arcing events.

2. *Reduce Your EMR Emissions and Exposure while You Sleep*

Sleep at least several feet from your circuit breaker panel. Whether it's off or on, it receives electricity from your neighborhood transformer and generates electromagnetic fields, including through walls.

Do not sleep near a wall that has a circuit breaker panel, a transmitting utility meter or a refrigerator on its other side.

Unplug the electronic devices in and near your bedroom while you sleep. Don't just turn off your TV, computer, and alarm clock: unplug them. Unplug all electric cords to devices around your bed and to the wall behind your bed. If you must have an alarm clock, get a battery operated one.

Never sleep with a mobile or DECT phone on or charging nearby. Exposure to RF fields decreases the secretion and effectiveness of melatonin, which is necessary for sound sleep—and cancer prevention.

Eliminate baby monitors, which commonly transmit microwaves.

Turn Wi-Fi off whenever you don't use it, especially at night. If you're not sure how to turn off your Wi-Fi, unplug the power to your computer, printer, and modem.

Do not sleep with an electric blanket or heating pad, or on a water bed.

In his book *Earthing*, Clint Ober reports on the numerous benefits of sleeping connected to the Earth. He sells conductive sheets and other products at his website. *Note*: If you have magnetic or electric fields in your bedroom, sleeping on conductive cloth that's plugged into an outlet may increase your exposure to those fields.[3] If you cannot eliminate the electrical field in your home, your best bet may be to unplug all electronics in your bedroom while you sleep.

3. Continue Reducing Your Emissions and Exposure

Do not allow a "smart" utility meter at your home, school, or office. If you've already got one (or more), get it off. Educate your neighbors about the hazards of transmitting meters, and

3 M. Virnich and M. Schauer, "Caution, Ground Pads and Sheets: Being Grounded is Not Equal to Zero-Field Exposure," *de–Der Elektro- und Gebäudetechniker* (11-2005) transl. by Katharina Gustavs, 2009.

encourage them to keep their analog meter (see Elizabeth Kelley's and Jerry Day's pieces in the appendix).

Eliminate fluorescent lights.[4] While they save energy, fluorescent lights require electronic ballasts (SMPSs), which generate square waves and harmonics. Their flickering can disturb the nervous system. Also, fluorescent bulbs are made with mercury, which is highly toxic if the bulb breaks. (Dispose of fluorescents at a special recycling facility.) LED bulbs have long life and use minimal electricity, but many styles also generate high frequencies. Try CLEDs, which don't require conversion from DC to AC. Stock up on incandescent bulbs, since manufacturing of them is being phased out. For big box stores and gymnasiums, consider 12-volt DC LEDs, *not* halogens with SMPSs. For more about flicker sensitivity, see conradbiologic.com.

Find non-electric ways to decorate your home during holidays.

Eliminate dimmer switches (which require SMPSs); *replace them with on/off switches.* If you want mood lighting, use lights with three levels.

Have an electrician rewire lights controlled by multiple switches so that all but one switch is disconnected. (Improperly installed, multiple switches can generate magnetic fields.)

Be aware that many large-screen TVs can create high frequency fields even throughout a large room.

Eliminate DECT phones. Use only corded landlines. DECT base stations emit RF signals. Find non-electric, corded landline phones at thrift shops and office supply stores. Some speakerphones do not require plugging into an electrical outlet.

Get cabled Internet access. Make sure the wireless transmitter in your cable box is turned off.

---

4 M. Havas, "Health concerns associated with energy efficient lighting and their electromagnetic emissions," *Scientific Committee on Emerging and Newly Identified Health Risks*, 2008.

If you can, live in a free-standing home. Sharing a wall increases your chance of exposure to magnetic fields and RF fields. Apartment dwellers whose outside wall holds "smart" meters are especially vulnerable.

Give your windows attention. In some houses (i.e., stucco, brick, and concrete), windows may be the main entry point for RF fields. Note: Using wireless devices within a house with low-energy transfer windows, aluminum siding, metal roofing, or metal window screens can intensify EMR exposure. Also, RF signals can pass through newer low-energy transfer windows. Aluminum screens and older low-energy transfer windows may block RF signals significantly—but not totally. Monitor your home for magnetic fields and RF fields regularly.

Eliminate furniture and carpets made from synthetic fiber, and replace them with materials that are less likely to become electro-statically charged.

To shield a room, you might try applying heat-controlled window film on the windows, shielding paint, and/or shielding fabric on the walls. Shielding is tricky, because some microwaves can penetrate some metal (i.e., cell phone signals can reach inside a car); and blocking microwaves from one direction can intensify the ones coming from another direction. Monitor the area frequently with quality meters, since new equipment can be installed nearby without your knowledge. Note that shielding microwaves will not shield you from EMFs.

⌘

Dan Stih, author of *Healthy Living Spaces: The Top Ten Hazards Affecting Your Health*, aerospace engineer: *If you feel sick in your house and suspect a wiring problem, a building biologist can help you identify what's wrong and describe it in a way that an electrician can understand and respect. If you live in an apartment complex or near an antenna, shielding paint or curtains can be* *worthwhile, and a building biologist can speed up your learning curve so that you use them properly. Meanwhile, for most people, I recommend prudent avoidance of wireless devices.*

ꕤ

Gary Olhoeft, PhD geophysicist and electrical engineer: *I bought a spectrum analyzer in order to regularly survey my house for dangerous levels of electromagnetic fields. I've learned where there are concentrations of energies in my house, and I avoid them. I know my bedroom is clean now.*

Most schools, libraries, malls, restaurants, courts, hospitals and other public places now have Wi-Fi. Many of these buildings also have bad grounds. Many newer cars come with built-in cell phones, Bluetooth and Wi-Fi—not to mention computerized, RF signal-emitting ignition systems. Some electric cars and hybrids' charging systems can create dirty power.

The FCC protects the spectrum bands of electrical devices. But it does not test everything—like fluorescent lights and TVs—or provide regulations or warnings about them. The FCC needs to warn people about what happens when more than one device operates in a room or a building. We also need a government agency that requires testing and disclosure of emissions of all electronic devices.

4. *Pregnant Women, Infants, and Children Should Not Use Wireless Devices*

A baby's developing brain is especially susceptible to radiation. If a pregnant woman uses a cell phone once per day, the chance of her child's developing behavioral problems nearly doubles, even after correcting for other effects.[5] If a pregnant woman

5 Divan et al, "Prenatal and postnatal exposure to cell phone use and behavioral problems in children," *Epidemiology*, vol. 19, no. 4 (2008) 523–529.

has an emergency and must use a cell phone, she should keep it away from her abdomen. No one should speak or text on a mobile phone while holding the device near a baby's head.

If you intend to conceive, *eliminate wireless devices before you start trying.*

A man who plans to become a father should not keep a cell phone in his pocket or on his belt. Keep cell phones turned off, since their use negatively affects sperm quality.[6] Studies about the effects of carrying a mobile phone on women's reproductive health have not been conducted; but women might apply the Precautionary Principle here.

Educate your children. Except for emergencies, children should not use mobile phones. The hazards of exposure to RF signals emitted by mobile devices are greater for children than they are for adults (see the American Academy of Pediatrics' letter in the appendices).

Schools should designate rooms with cabled Internet access for students and teachers who choose them.

If you teach, invite students to learn their phones' SAR levels at different settings, with and without a Bluetooth, at different distances. Have each student create their own safety standards for using a mobile device, and compare them to the standards set by the FCC, the BioInitiative Report and the Seletun Statement.

⌘

Liz Bateman, 27, Southeast: *Recently, I spent a day on a train and was nauseous the whole time. I've ridden trains before and never had a problem. A friend wondered if the train's new Wi-Fi system might have affected me.*

---

6 G. N. De Iuliis et al, "Mobile phone radiation induces reactive oxygen species production and DNA damage in human spermatozoa in vitro," *PLoS One*, vol. 4, no. 7 (2009): e6446.

I had no idea that Wi-Fi could be harmful. But I realized that my depression and a sinus infection that would not quit started around the time my husband and I got cell phones and Wi-Fi. As I learned more, I felt unsafe talking on the cell phone. My husband and I want children, and we want them to have a healthy start. We decided to go back to a corded landline and cabled Internet access. This actually took two months, including a five-hour "conversation" with our phone company and a week without a phone. We kept a cell phone for emergencies.

Remarkably, my husband and I now feel less anxious. And since we're not always available to each other, we actually communicate more clearly.

5. If You Use a Cell Phone or any Other Mobile Device

Keep it off. The phone emits pulses of microwave radiation regularly to antennas whenever it can send or receive texts or calls. Therefore, keep Airplane mode turned on. Or, remove the phone's battery. Install the battery only when you use the phone.

Avoid using a mobile phone in elevators, airplanes, busses, trains, and subways since it exposes you and others in your vicinity to EMFs.[7]

Start with a Tech Sabbath. One day each week, do not use a cell phone or a mobile device, and see if your health or sleep changes.

Create "no-device zones" in your kitchen and dining room and in your car, as psychologist Sherry Turkle (author of *Alone Together*) suggests.

Follow guidelines suggested by the American Academy of Pediatrics ("Children, Adolescents and the Media," issued on 12.28.13): Do not allow children under two any media exposure. Do not allow devices with screens in children's bedrooms.

7 R. Herberman, "Practical Advice to Limit Exposure to Electromagnetic Radiation Emitted from Cell Phones"; environmentaloncology.org /node/202 (7-2008).

Filters

A properly designed filter may reduce magnetic fields, the amplitude of high frequencies, or RF electromagnetic radiation. No filter can eliminate a *source* of dirty power. Different kinds of electrical problems require different kinds of filters (i.e., ferrites, inductors, and pi filters). Some problems may not respond to filtering. Effective filters may cost $1/watt.

Some filters have capacitors that reduce the amplitude of some high frequencies on power lines. Note that filters with capacitors consume electricity. Also, if a filter is plugged in behind a bed, say, the magnetic field at the bed may actually increase. Some companies make medical filters (i.e., that shield EEG machines) and military filters.

ꕤ

Gary Olhoeft, PhD, geophysicist and electrical engineer: *As a geophysicist, I had a lab for testing soil affected by pesticides and other chemicals. Signals emitted by the elevator in my building and by a nearby machine shop interfered with my extremely sensitive meters. In order to work, I outfitted my lab (at significant expense) with active operational amplifier filters. They can reduce everything below one MHz that comes in on power lines to outlets in a building. As radiofrequencies became more ubiquitous because of Wi-Fi and other signals, I shielded the walls (again at significant expense) with aluminum and permalloy.*

Graham-Stetzer filters were designed in the early 2000s to reduce high frequencies that ride on 60 Hz wires—i.e., conducted radiation, not induced or radiated parts of dirty power. Some people find Graham-Stetzer filters beneficial. Others find that they aggravate their symptoms. Among people who seek solutions for dirty power, Stetzer filters can be a contentious issue (Electricalpollution.com endorses Stetzer filters; emfrelief.com/capacitive-filters.html and conradbiologic.com/articles/emfscams.html; post info about why Stetzer filters [different from the operational amplitude filters that Gary Olhoeft describes] may aggravate symptoms).

ꕥ

Jessie Grant, 38, Northwest: *I have several friends whose EHS symptoms decreased when they installed Stetzer filters. I've tried Graham-Stetzer and Green Wave filters in two houses, and each time I plugged them in, I felt like someone planted a trail of splinters along my spine.*

ꕥ

Michael Schwaebe, mechanical engineer and building biology environmental consultant, California: *When Stetzer filters are installed in a home or building with concurrent wiring errors (e.g., multipath current returns), magnetic fields are exacerbated. The filters change electrical transient "noise" to current—e.g., volts to amps. Each filter adds about one amp to the current flow in that circuit. If there's a multi-path return, then the current flows are not equal and opposite in all of the loops. This causes magnetic fields to elevate. For people with sensitivity to electric fields, symptoms may be reduced. For people with sensitivity to subtle magnetic fields, symptoms may be aggravated, even when the wiring is correct.*

Do not use mobile phones or tablets to send or receive pictures or movies—technology that requires more bandwidth. Use only *wired* computers to send or receive pictures and movies.

⌘

Ginger Farver: *If mobile phone users ask me how to protect themselves from exposure to electromagnetic radiation, I suggest they start by following the guidelines in their cell phone's manual. Many manufacturers suggest keeping the phone at least nine tenths of an inch away from your body, and that pregnant women and teenagers should keep phones away from their lower abdomens.*

Limit mobile phone calls to emergencies, and keep them short. Using a mobile phone for thirty minutes a day is the heaviest use studied so far, and it significantly increases your risk of brain cancer.[8]

Do not use a laptop or pad on your lap or near internal organs.

Be aware: the weaker an antenna's signal, the more your cell phone has to increase its radiation output to maintain the connection with the relay antenna, which increases your exposure. Swedish research finds worse health effects for cell phone users in rural areas, where reception is poor.

If your ear feels warm, end the call immediately.

Use a corded microphone and earbuds and keep the phone away from your body. Do not use a cordless (Bluetooth) earpiece, which is just another radio too close to your head. Text or use the speakerphone.

Don't text or phone in a metal box such as an elevator, car, bus or train, since this also requires your phone to increase

8 E. Cardis et al, "Brain tumor risk in relation to mobile telephone use: Results of the INTERPHONE international case controlled study," *International Journal of Epidemiology*, vol 39, no. 3 (2010): 675–694.

its radiation output. People in the metal box will receive this increased radiation. Children and people with medical implants could be significantly impacted.

Don't text or talk while driving. Texting or talking on a mobile phone while driving is illegal in many states and more dangerous than driving drunk, even with a hands-free device. To quote a bumper sticker from NorthSun.com: *If you want to see God, keep texting while you drive.*

Beware of gizmos. A trinket on your neck or phone can't block microwaves. Air tube headsets are safer; but you need to keep the phone as far away from you as possible while you use it. If you have an emergency and must use a phone, use it in speakerphone mode.

Kindly ask guests to keep mobile phones in their cars or to place them inside a covered metal pot while they visit. Inside a covered metal pot, a mobile phone cannot transmit or receive signals.

Be aware that no study has explored the combined effects of exposure to magnetic fields, cell phones, Wi-Fi, "smart" meters, and the risk of cancers below the neck, including leukemia, lymphoma, skin and pancreatic cancers.

Detox gently. This means changing habits and detoxing over the long term, rather than over a weekend.

6. Educate Others and Take Political Action

I've found that if I am even minimally angry or irritated when I talk about the health or environmental effects of mobile devices, Wi-Fi, antennas, and "smart" meters, my efforts can be ineffective or even harmful.

Indeed, sharing information about this stuff is tricky. Many people find the idea that their mobile phones and Wi-Fi can harm them or others ludicrous and offensive. Speaking in a "neutral" tone that allows the person on the other side of my conversation space for their own thoughts and emotions requires a kind of sainthood that, frankly, I don't often have, especially while I perceive that the whole planet is at stake.

Studies show that if a person believes an idea (i.e., mobile phones are safe), then hears it contradicted (i.e., mobile phones are *not* safe), they will probably attach more strongly than ever to the first idea.

If I approach any situation thinking that *I* know what another person needs to do, I offend them.

Once, living in a townhouse, I wrote my neighbors a letter explaining that because of a health condition, my doctor recommends that I reduce my exposure to electromagnetic radiation. I wondered if they could turn their Wi-Fi and mobile phones off at night. These people were so offended that they reported my request to our neighborhood association. They need Wi-Fi to stay competitive, they need their mobile phones available 24/7 to family—and their devices are all FCC approved.

Yikes! My letter (which seemed polite and logical to me) only widened the gap between us.

How do we create options for everyone in our communities while some perceive that they cannot survive without wireless devices—and others perceive that wireless devices threaten our entire ecosystem? Can I respect people who love mobile devices, even when children are involved?

Effective activists tell me that successful projects start by gathering people and naming what we agree on.

Flyers (i.e., about the dangers of "smart" meters or proposed antennas) are most effective when they present *minimal* information. The less words on the page, the greater the chance they'll get read.

If you're asked to give an educational talk about wireless devices, show one of the DVDs listed in the resource section so you don't have to reinvent the wheel. Follow the movie with a Q&A session. Ideally, the panelists who respond to questions are well-versed in your local situation and can explain complex things (like the Telecom Act and studies about the non-thermal effects of RF signals) *briefly.*

Inform Yourself and Your Neighbors

A first step: *Ask and listen.* Ask neighbors if they've noticed changes in their sleep, anxiety levels, skin, memory, headaches, or other symptoms since "smart" meters, cellular antennas, and/or upgrades to antennas were installed in your area. Just listen to their reports. Read Elizabeth Kelley's suggestions in the appendix. Assemble a neighborhood study and action group. Another initial step: *Go to antennasearch.com* and learn how many antennas are within a four-mile radius of your home, school, or workplace.

Alert owners about antennas' negative effects on property values *before* they contract with a telecom company.

Learn about your town's telecom ordinance. Many ordinances allow telecom companies to install antennas on easements to private property without notice or permission. To learn more, refer to *Cell Towers: State of the Science/State of the Law*, edited by B. Blake Levitt. Check out the Coalition for Local Oversight of Utility Technologies; www.CLOUTnow.org.

If you write a letter to your newspaper, get at least three people to edit your piece for tone (may it respect wireless service subscribers), *accuracy* (about electricity and RF fields, studies, and telecom policy), and *good grammar.*

Respectfully alert friends and neighbors who are dismayed by corporate control that telecom companies have more lobbyists than the oil and health insurance industries. How to deal with this? Telecom companies' funding comes from people who subscribe to their services.

Divest. If you own telecom stock or subscribe to wireless services, divest.

Petition Congressional Representatives to Sponsor Legislation such as:

The Cell Phone Right to Know Act, 2012 HR6358, which would require telecom companies to share their records for health research, the EPA to revise safety standards on mobile devices every two years, and SAR labeling on cell phones. Electricalpollution.com has a sample letter to send your legislators.

Whitney North Seymour Jr.'s amendment to Section 704 of The Telecommunications Act of 1996. Currently, Section 704 prevents state or local governments from regulating the placement, construction, or modification of telecom equipment based on the environmental effects of radio frequency emissions. Mr. Seymour's amendment would restore local governments' ability to make zoning decisions that protect their citizens' general welfare. If you'd like to petition your legislator to sponsor this amendment, please contact emrpolicy.org; in the subject header, write "Amend 704."

Petition Your School Board and School Administrators

Get your town's public and private schools to ban Wi-Fi. To begin, refer to recommendations in "Autism and EMF? Plausibility of a pathophysiological link—parts 1 and 2" by Dr. Martha Herbert (pediatric neurologist at Harvard Medical School) and Cindy Sage (coeditor of the BioInitiative Reports) in *Pathophysiology* 2013.[9]

When telecom companies offer rent to keep antennas on poorly funded school grounds, administrators and parents often have no idea about the hazards of such equipment.[10]

Citizens for Safe Technology offers concerned parents a Wi-Fi non-consent form that educates adults in a school community about Wi-Fi and children's health (c4st.org).

---

9 See safeschool.ca; Wi-Fiinschools.org.uk; or wiredchild.org.

10 See www.centerforsaferwireless.org/Cell-Phone-Towers-and-Antennas-on-School-Property.php.

Dr. Magda Havas's BRAG (TM) Antenna Ranking of Schools (based on the proximity and density of antennas near schools), teaches parents how to BRAG Rate their children's school if it is not listed (magdahavas.com/wordpress/wp-content/uploads/2010/04/BRAG_How-to.pdf).

⚭

Denise Barker, 32: *When I learned that my children's elementary school plans to install Wi-Fi, I prepared a series of lectures for parents and teachers to learn about the hazards of wireless devices. I distributed letters on the subject by Dr. Martha Herbert and the American Academy of Pediatrics. At wifiinschools.org.uk, Dr. Sarah Starkey lists scientific studies that demonstrate the impact of RF radiation on DNA, sleep, fertility, behavior, melatonin and more.*

Several parents and teachers told me that they question these studies. They've seen Wi-Fi enhance many children's interest in school. I felt so discouraged that I almost canceled the lectures. Then I realized I need to meet others who do not want Wi-Fi in our school. Even if I only connect with one other person, I need to meet!

Report Problems

If a device makes you sick, report the problem to the FDA's Medwatch Program, www.accessdata.fda.gov/scripts/medwatch/medwatch-online.htm or 800.FDA.1088. Report it to the Consumer Product Safety Commission, which takes dangerous products off the market: 800.638.2772 or cpsc.gov/cgibin/incident.aspx. File complaints about wireless devices limiting your ability to work, frequent public space or find healthy housing with the ADA *and* with the Justice Department's civil rights division. Send a copy of your complaints to info@emrpolicy.org with "Radiation Emitting Product Complaint" in the subject heading and to *Consumer Reports*.

Petition Your State's Legislators

Get your state to designate an energy-efficient, energy and chemically safe, radio-free zone. Such zones would have no transmitting utility meters, Wi-Fi, mobile phones, cellular antennas, or cordless landlines. Internet connections would be cabled. Pesticides and other hazardous chemicals would not be allowed.

⌘

Jody McLaughlin, 57, Washington: *I find it ironic that in my search for a place with minimal RF radiation, I tell people that I'm looking for a dead zone.*

Be gentle with thyself. These issues are massive, and we are mere mortals. Remember that small steps can accumulate into significant change. Recognizing that we've made mistakes in regulating and using electricity and wireless devices is a big step. So is asking questions: *Would I rather have more technology or live within my biological limitations? What can I do?*

12

Closing Questions

The electronic technologies that we now depend on may well put life as we know it at risk. *What would Rachel Carson suggest?* In concluding *Silent Spring*, Carson observed that those who manufactured and used pesticides possessed "no humility before the vast forces with which they tamper."

Does our species' survival depend on humbling ourselves? Could we admit how much we do not understand about the things we've depended on since birth; how much we have taken electricity, appliances, electronics, and telecommunications for granted? Could we recognize that our technological advances harm our health and wildlife health? Could we each acknowledge our electronic footprints?

The longer any individual, family, community, or country ignores the dangers of radiation emitted by electronics and wireless devices, the more severe the consequences.

What do we need to achieve a constructive discussion? What actions will reduce our emissions of and exposure to electromagnetic radiation? What will keep us in discussion so that the coming Spring is not silent?

Appendices

Resources

Legal and Regulatory Issues

Levitt, B. Blake, *Electromagnetic Fields: A Consumer's Guide to the Issues and How to Protect Ourselves*, Harcourt Brace, 1996.

Steneck, N.H., ed., *Risk/Benefit Analysis: The Microwave Case*, San Francisco Press, 1982.

www.emrpolicy.org; tracks scientific and public policy developments in the EMR health debate.

www.antennasearch.com; lists licensed antennas within four miles of a given address.

www.commlawblog.com/2013/04/articles/cellular/fcc-looks-at-health-effects-of-radio-waves/index.html.

www.bit.ly/1aGxQiq posts; comments filed to the FCC between June 24 and November 18, 2013 regarding its cell phone radiation regulations.

www.international-emf-alliance.org; lists groups that call for stricter regulation and/or a moratorium on wireless technologies.

Scientific Studies about EMR

Bioelectromagnetism: Principles and Applications, 2nd edition, J. Malmivuo and Robert Plonsey, Oxford U. Press, 2013.

On the Nature of Electromagnetic Field Interactions with Biological Systems, Allan Frey, ed., Landes Co., 1994.

Pathophysiology, Aug. 2009 (special issue devoted to EMR and health, edited by cell biologist Martin Blank, PhD).

Physics Today, March 2013 (special issue dedicated to new discoveries such as bioelectric signaling controlling tissue shape and structure).

Warnke, Ulrich, *Bees, Birds and Mankind: Effects of Wireless Communication Technologies,* Kentum, 2009.

www.bioinitiative.org; *The BioInitiative 2012 Report.* 1800 peer-reviewed studies about effects of magnetic fields and RF radiation since 2007 on fertility, autism, DNA, childhood cancers, breast cancer, Alzheimer's, and the nervous system. Check out the RF Color Charts, which list more than 50 key studies of the biological effects of low-intensity exposure *and* exposure standards set by IEEE and FCC.

www.emfacts.com/electricwords; an index of scientific studies.

www.emf-portal.de; includes studies about mold and EMR.

www.magdahavas.com/category/from-zorys-archive/; studies on the health effects of RF radiation exposure conducted before 1975.

www.microwavenews.com; longtime watchdog of the telecom industry.

www.moef.nic.in/downloads/public-information/final_mobile_towers_report.pdf; posts the Report on Possible Impacts of Communication Towers on Wildlife Including Birds and Bees, commissioned by India's Ministry of Environment and Forests.

General Information

Crofton, Kerry, PhD, *Wireless Radiation Rescue*, Global Wellbeing Books, 2010. Includes excellent resources.

Davis, Devra, *Disconnect: The Truth About Cell Phone Radiation, What the Industry is Doing to Hide It, and How to Protect Your Family*, Dutton, 2010.

Keithley, John, *The Story of Electrical and Magnetic Measurements from 500 BC to the 1940s*, Wiley-IEEE, 1999.

Turkle, Sherry, *Alone Together: Why We Expect More From Technology and Less From Each Other*, Basic Books, 2011.

www.electronicsilentspring.com; has intro packets about key issues and updates this book.
www.emfsafetynetwork.org; posts "smart" meter health complaints, advocacy support, ideas for parents and more.
www.centerforsaferwireless.org; focuses on EMR and health.
www.c4st.ca; Canadians for Safe Technology.
www.electromagnetichealth.org; "Cell Phones and Brain Tumors."
www.electricalpollution.com; posts notice about govt. calls for comments on proposed changes to EMR emmissions standards.
www.es-uk.info; based in UK.
www.mastsanity.org; info about EMR's environmental effects.
www.mast-victims.org; stories from people harmed by antennas.
www.powerwatch.org.uk; longtime British site.

"Smart" Meters

At freedomtaker.com, Jerry Day offers a letter you can send to your utility company to demand *removal* of a transmitting meter and a (replacement) analog meter. A man whose pacemaker shut off after "smart" meters were installed in his neighborhood speaks on a video. See the appendix for Jerry Day's model letter that refuses *installation* of a "smart" meter.

Sage Associates, environmental consultants, offers "Thirteen Fatal Flaws of Smart Meter Technology" and "Assessment of Radio frequency Microwave Radiation Emissions from 'smart' meters" at sagereports.com.

Independent researcher Ronald M. Powell, PhD in applied physics from Harvard, has an excellent paper, "Biological effects from RF radiation at low-intensity exposure, based on the BioInitiative 2012 report and the implications for 'smart' meters and smart appliances," available at emfsafetynetwork.org.

Industrial Hygienist Peter H. Sierck's "Smart Meters: What Do We Know? A Technical Paper to Clarify RF Radiation Emissions and Measurement Methodologies," at www.EMFRF.com, presents a way of scientifically measuring the strength of microbursts emitted by "smart" meters and how frequently microbursts occur. It summarizes concerns and presents options if you have had a "smart" meter installed.

Electrical engineer Tom Wilson speaks about the health and environmental risks of the "smart" grid at the Wireless Safety Summit in October, 2011; posted at www.youtube /com/watch?feature=player_embedded&v=YPoLvTNRxhs. An accompanying power point is at www.s4ar.com/smart _meter_wireless_safety_summit_Power_Pointe.pdf and at electromagneticsafety.org under "Expert Opinions."

Engineer Rob States has a video on YouTube called "The Dark Side of 'smart' meters."

"Smart Metering Projects Map" shows a global picture of deployment; https://maps.google.com/mapsms?ie=UTF8 &oe=UTF8&msa=0&msid=115519311058367343480 .00000113 62ac6d7d21187.

"Take Back Your Power," Josh del Sol's film about "smart" meters; TakeBackYourPower.net.

www.emfsafetynetwork.org; the EMF Safety Network launched the (now international) campaign against "smart" meters in Sebastopol, California, in 2009. The site posts many important compilations, including "Smart Meter Fires and Explosions."

www.smartmeterdangers.org.

www.stopsmartmeters.org.

www.smartmeterlock.com; locks that prevent removal of analog meters.

⌘

Alex Richards, tech executive and entrepreneur: *Supposedly, "smart" meters were installed for utility companies to know when consumers use computers, battery chargers, hot tubs—and to suggest tips for changing usage times and saving money. What if the companies just gave us these tips? Instead of meters that continuously pulse and emit radiation, could we get analog meters that send data to the utility company for one minute per month? Or, could subscribers send a monthly* *reading to the utility company via the Internet, the telephone or snail mail?*

EMR and Health

The Austrian Medical Association posts guidelines on diagnosis and treatment of EMF-related health problems at www.aerztekammer.at/documents/10618/976981/EMF-Guideline.pdf.

Black and White: Voices and Witnesses About Electro-Hyper-Sensitivity: The Swedish Experience, compiled by Rigmor Granlund-Lind and John Lind, at feb.se/feb/blackonwhite-complete-book.pdf.

Becker, Robert O., MD, *The Body Electric: Electromagnetism and the Foundation of Life,* William Morrow, 1985.

Becker, Robert O., MD, *Cross Currents: The Perils of Electropollution*, Tarcher, 1990.

Brodeur, Paul, *The Zapping of America: Microwaves, Their Deadly Rise and Coverup*, WW Norton, 1977.

www.feb.se From Sweden, the first advocacy for electrosensitive people.

www.healthandhabitat.com Posted by Sandra Ross, MD, about reducing EMFs in hospitals and medical offices.

www.heartmdinstitute.com/v1/wireless-safety/cordless-phone-use-can-affect-heart shows cardiologist Stephen Sinatra, MD explaining why radiation from wireless devices cause cell inflammation, heart disease and more.

Medical Implants

Dr. Gary Olhoeft speaks about "Electromagnetic Interference and Medical Implants" at www.youtube/com/results?search_query=olhoeft&sm=12.

www.fda.gov/MedicalDevices/.

Francis, J., and M. Niehaus, "Interference between cellular telephones and implantable rhythm devices: A review on recent papers:" *Indian Pacing and Electrophysiology Journal,* vol. 6, no. 4 (2006): p 226–233.

Halperin, D. et al, "Pacemakers and implantable cardiac defibrillators: Software radio attacks and zero-power defenses," *IEEE Symposium on Security and Privacy.*

Sutter, J. D., "Scientists work to keep hackers out of implanted medical devices, CNN, 4-16-2010.

Talan, Jamie, *Deep Brain Stimulation*, Dana Press, 2009.

youtube.com/watch?v=brdhogkdxw4 shows a video of a man whose pacemaker shut off after a "smart" meter was installed on his property.

Ideas, Meters, Filters, Shielding Products, and Tools with Fewer EMFs

www.buildingbiology.ca Includes building biology consultant Katharina Gustavs' 2008 paper, "Options to Minimize Non-Ionizing Electromagnetic Radiation Exposures (EMF /RF/Static Fields) in Office Environments."

For filters that comply with international standards as well as shielding from power surges caused by lightning and construction and ferrites that clamp on a cable to absorb conducted RF riding on the outside of a wire, see cor.com (847.680.7400); Curtis Industries (800-657-0853); leadertechinco.com (813-855-6921); schurterinc.com (707-636-3000) and Environmental Potentials at ep2000.com (800-500-7536). Some of these businesses also provide shielding for individual computers, circuit boards, and air vents.

www.lehmans.org; non-electric tools and appliances.

www.lessemfs.org; meters, shielding products, books and DVDs.

www.magneticsciences.com (978-266-9355); sells and rents meters for magnetic fields, RFs and more. Serves homeowners, academic researchers, people with medical implants, and industry.

www.safelivingtechnologies.ca; sells meters, shielding paint and fabric.

Energy and Mineral Issues

Cook, Gary, "How Green Is Your Cloud?" The Greenpeace Policy Analyst describes data centers visible from space and that require as much energy to operate as it takes to power 250,000 European homes. Greenpeace.org

Glanz, James, "Power, Pollution and the Internet: Industry Wastes Vast Amounts of Electricity, Belying Image," 9-23-12, *NY Times*.

Pariser, Eli, *The Filter Bubble: What the Internet is Hiding from You*, Penguin, 2011.

Simpson, Cam, "The Deadly Tin Inside Your Smartphone," *Businessweek*, August 23, 2012.

www.electronicstakeback.com/toxics-in-electronics/.

Privacy Issues

www.eff.org/issues/privacy The Electronic Frontier Foundation.

Wi-Fi in Schools

"Autism and EMF? Plausibility of a pathophysiological link—Parts I and II," by Dr. Martha Herbert (pediatric neurologist at Harvard) and Cindy Sage, MA (coeditor of the *BioInitiative Report*), in *Pathophysiology* 2013; for a recorded conversation with Dr. Herbert and Cindy Sage, see healthandenvironment.org/wg~calls/13091.

emfsafetynetwork.org; posts a two-minute video of Professor Olle Johansson warning of wireless DNA damage to children *and* "Is Wi-Fi Safe?"

EMRPolicy.org has an excellent page dedicated to Wi-Fi in schools (see EMRPolicy.org/public~policy/schools/index .htm).

www.saferemr.com/2013_03_01_archive.html posts eight experts' letters, submitted to the Los Angeles Unified School District while it considered installing Wi-Fi.

http://youtu.be/GJPTzaNkcUk; posts a ten minute video about wireless precaution in Australian schools.

http://wifiinschools.com/; a consumer advocacy site.

http://wifiinschools.org.uk/resources/safeschools2012.pdf; posts "Safe Schools 2012," medical experts call for safe technologies in schools.

Links for Teens

In Germany, teachers can borrow a "phantom head" that measures cell-phone radiation emissions and Specific Absorption Rates so that students can learn exactly the radiation their phones deliver; www.maschek.de/uk/frameset.php?p=produkte.

The International Commission on Electromagnetic Safety has a webpage for teens and cell phone safety, which includes links to four videos; www.iceems.eu/public_education.htm.

"Cell Phones: Teens in the Driver's Seat," at youtube.com/watch?v=1SrFqhqfZ5Y.

"Cell Phones: Just Like Cigarettes?" at youtube.com/watch?v=XIPtEYIOupE.

"Expert EMF Workshop at San Leandro High School," Moderated by Ari Dolid, a teacher and advisor to the student-led Social Justice Academy, and Elizabeth Kelley, Director of ICEMS. Includes presentations by Dr. Magda Havas, Dr. Henry Lai and Dr. Raymond Neutra.

"Small Group Discussion: Safer Cell Phone Use," an informal conversation between experts and students.

See http://Wi-Fiinschools.org/uk/; www.centerforsaferwireless.org/Educational-Materials-for-Teens-Using-Cell-Phones.php.

Radio-free Zones

Around the world, a few radio-free zones have been established. In Europe, several are designed for electrically-hypersensitive people. Others occur second-handedly around government-operated astronomy stations. (To prevent interference with sensitive telescopes, nearby residents and visitors may be severely restricted from using wireless devices.) Several refuges have closed after antennas were installed nearby.

In Greenbank, West Virginia, the National Radio Astronomy Observatory prohibits anything that produces RF fields, including satellites and wireless devices. Some electrically-sensitive people find their symptoms eased in Greenbank; others find them aggravated.

The Murchison Radio-astronomy Observatory in western Australia has a radio-quiet zone: www.atnf.csiro.au/projects/askap/ASKAP_FAQ_Pastoralists_March2012.pdf.

WIRES (Women's Initiative to Reduce Electro Smog) has begun investigating the possibility of creating a radio free zone in Ontario, Canada on Lake Huron. Along with a city planner, WIRES is exploring what limits might be imposed on residents. For example, would microwave ovens be allowed? How/could limits be enforced?

In Europe, small radio-free zones have been designated around astronomy stations in Belgium, Czech Republic, Finland, and France. In November 2011, Sweden's Dalarna County began preparing to create a radiation-free zone because one of its residents is electrosensitive.

For a refuge in France, go to www.ehs-refuge-zone.eu.

To minimize exposure to magnetic fields, look for towns with a Delta electrical system and no transmitting utility meters.

To minimize exposure to cellular antenna RF fields, go to antennasearch.com for info about a specific address. Electromagnetichealth.org recommends hilly, mountainous regions where cell phone reception isn't easily accessed. Look at telecom companies' coverage maps to identify areas with no or few antennas:

www.verizonwireless.com/b2c/support/coverage-locator.
www.wireless.att.com/coverageviewer/.
www.coverage.spring.com/.
www.t-mobile.com/coverage/pcc.aspx.
www.boostmobile.com/coverage/.
www.mycricket.com/coverage/maps/wireless.
www.virginmobileusa.com/check-cell-phone-coverage.
www.uscellular.com/maps.
www.maps.metropcs.com.
www.tracfone.com/cellular_coverage.jsp.

DVDs

Congressional Staff Briefing About Wireless and Broadcast Radiation Pollution given in May, 2007 from environmental consultant Cindy Sage, attorney Deb Carney, Whitney N. Seymour, Jr. (cofounder of the Natural Resources Defense Council, former U.S. Attorney General for NY's Southern District), Dr. Albert Manville (U.S. Fish & Wildlife), Dr. Martin Blank (biophysicist at Columbia U.), Blake Levitt (former science writer for the *NY Times)*. Available from emrpolicy.org.

Full Signal, filmmaker Talal Jabari, 2009. Citizens, scientists and doctors from eight countries discuss cell phones, antennas, and health.

Public Exposure: DNA, Democracy and the Wireless Revolution, produced by the Council on Wireless Technology Impacts (energyfields.org) and Ecological Options Network (eon3 .net), 2007. Presents the telecom industry's cover-up of dangers posed by cell phones and antennas. Includes a Congressional staff briefing by physicist Ted Litovitz about how EMR affects living organisms (also available at electromagnetichealth.org).

Resonance: Beings of Frequency, James Russell's film describes how birds, bees, and people have adapted over millions of years to the Earth's electromagnetic energy—and how exposure to human-made frequencies challenges our health and survival. vimeo.com/54189727.

Take Back Your Power, Josh del Sol's film about the "smart" grid; thepowerfilm.org.

Magazine Articles

"Danger Calling?" *Green American*, January, 2011.

"Cell-Phone Safety: What the FCC Didn't Test," by Michael Scherer, *Time*, October 26, 2010.

"Electro Shocker," by Michael Segell, *Prevention Magazine*, January, 2010. How dirty electricity created a cancer cluster at a California school.

"Warning: Your Cell Phone May Be Hazardous to Your Health," by Christopher Ketcham, *GQ*, February, 2010.

For Travelers

Be aware that a hotel or a neighboring building may have antennas on its rooftop. The antenna might be concealed to look like a chimney. Hotels have no obligation to inform guests about such installations. Therefore, *ask*.

If requested, a bed & breakfast may turn Wi-Fi off at night.

Consider camping. Some sites limit Wi-Fi to the concession area.

For hotels that use unscented cleaning products and provide cabled Internet connections, try puresolutions.com; 877-787-7666.

American Academy of Pediatrics

Dedicated to the Health of All Children
www.aap.org

December 12, 2012
The Honorable Dennis Kucinich
Rayburn House Office Building
Washington DC 20515

Dear Representative Kucinich:

On behalf of the American Academy of Pediatrics (AAP), a non-profit professional organization of 60,000 primary care pediatricians, pediatric medical sub-specialists, and pediatric surgical specialists dedicated to the health, safety and well-being of infants, children, adolescents, and young adults, I would like to share our support of H.R. 6358, the Cell Phone Right to Know Act.

The AAP strongly supports H.R. 6358's emphasis on examining the effects of radio frequency (RF) energy on vulnerable populations, including children and pregnant women. In addition, we are pleased that the bill would require the consideration of those effects when developing maximum exposure standards. Children are disproportionately affected by environmental exposures, including cell phone radiation. The differences in bone density and the amount of fluid in a child's brain compared to an adult's brain could allow children to absorb greater quantities of RF energy deeper into their brains than adults. It is essential that any new standards for cell phones or other wireless devices be based on protecting the youngest and most vulnerable populations to ensure they are safeguarded through their lifetimes.

In addition, the AAP supports the product labeling requirements of H.R. 6358. These standards will ensure consumers can make informed choices in selecting mobile phone purchases. They will also enable parents to better understand the potential dangers of RF energy exposure and protect their children.

On July 24, the U.S. Government Accountability Office (GAO) published a report on federal cell phone radiation exposure limits and testing requirements. The GAO noted that the Federal Communications Commission's (FCC) most recent data indicates that the number of estimated mobile phone subscribers has grown from approximately 3.5 million in 1989 to approximately 289 million at the end of 2009. Cell phone use behaviors have also changed during that time. The quantity and duration of cell phone calls has increased, as has the amount of times people use mobile phones, while cell phone and wireless technology has undergone substantial changes. Many people, especially adolescents and young adults, now use cell phones as their only phone line, and they begin using wireless phones at much younger ages.

Despite these dramatic changes in mobile phone technology and behavior, the FCC has not revisited the standard for cell phone radiation exposure since 1996. The current FCC standard for maximum radiation exposure levels is based on the heat emitted by mobile phones. These guidelines specify exposure limits for hand-held wireless devices in terms of the Specific Absorption Rate (SAR), which measures the rate the body absorbs radio frequency (RF). The current allowable SAR limit is 1.6 watts per kilogram (W/kg), as averaged over one gram of tissue. Although wireless devices sold in the United States must ensure that they do not exceed the maximum allowable SAR limit when operating at the device's highest possible power level, concerns have been raised that long-term RF energy exposure at this level affects the brain and other tissues and may be connected to types of brain cancer, including glioma and meningioma.

In May 2011, the International Agency for Research on Cancer (IARC), the United Nations' World Health Organization's (WHO) agency promoting international cancer research collaboration, classified RF energy as "possibly carcinogenic to humans." In addition, the National Cancer Institute has stated that although studies have not definitively linked RF energy exposure from cell phones to cancer, more research is required to address rapidly changing cell phone technology and use patterns.

This and other research identified by the GAO demonstrates the need for further research on this issue, and makes clear that exposure standards should be reexamined.

The GAO concluded that the current exposure limits may not reflect the latest research on RF energy, and that current mobile phone testing requirements may not identify maximum RF energy exposure. The GAO proposed that the FCC formally reassess its limit and testing requirements to determine whether they are effective. The AAP commends the activities proposed under H.R. 6358, as they would address the research gap and improve consumer knowledge and safety. Establishing an expanded federal research program as the basis for exposure standards will ensure that consumer protection incorporate the latest research. Currently, the National Institute of Health (NIH), the only federal agency the GAO identified as directly funding research on this topic, provided approximately $35 million from 2001 to 2011. Given this previous funding level, the AAP supports the $50 million per fiscal year for seven years that H.R. 6358 would authorize.

The AAP appreciates your recognition of the need for new research and standards for mobile phone radiation, and is pleased to support H.R. 6358.

Sincerely,
Thomas K. McInerny, MD, FAAP

Author's note: the FCC's revised standards, which reclassify the outer part of the ear as an extremity and thereby allow it a SAR of 4.0 W/kg over 10 g of tissue, went into effect in September, 2013.

De-Kun Li, MD, PhD, MPH, Senior Research Scientist Kaiser Permanente Division of Research, Oakland, CA[1]

Response to California Council on Science and Technology (CCST)

March 31, 2011

Dear Ms. Martin:

Thank you for inviting me to provide my professional opinions on the SmartMeter safety issue. I will address two questions raised in the attached letter. But first, here is some background information:

1. Currently there are no national or international "standards" for safety levels of radio frequency (a range of 3kHz to 300 GHz) devices. What FCC is currently using are "guidelines" which have much lower certainty than a "standard." One can go to many governmental agencies' websites like NIOSH, EPA, FDA, etc. to verify this. Therefore, for anyone to claim that they "meet FCC standards" gives a false impression of safety certainty compared to "guidelines," which implies that a lot is "unknown."
2. The current FCC "guideline was adopted by FCC based on EPA's recommendation in 1996. EPA made the recommendation "with certain reservation." There was a letter by Norbert Hankin, Center for Science and Risk Assessment, Radiation Protection Division at EPA, describing the current FCC guidelines. (The letter can be found through a Google search.) According to Hankin's letter, the FCC current guidelines were solely based on "thermal effects" of radio frequency, a level at which radio frequency can cause heat injury. As we know, heat injury is not what the public

1 See www.ccst.us/publications/2011/2011smartresources.php.

is concerned about regarding radio frequency safety. Their concerns are about cancer, miscarriages, birth defects, low semen quality, autoimmune disease, etc. Hankin's letter specifically emphasized that the EPA recommended guidelines that FCC is currently using do not apply to non-thermal effects of mechanisms (e.g., cancer, birth defects, miscarriage, autoimmune diseases, etc.) which are the focus of the public's concern. Hankin's letter states, "Therefore, the generalizations by many that the guidelines protect human beings from harm by any or all mechanisms is not justified."

3. In addition to being limited to only the thermal effect, the letter also states that the current FCC guidelines recommended by EPA were only based on experiments on animals in laboratories. Establishing firm safety standards usually requires evidence from human studies such as epidemiological studies. The current FCC guidelines were based on animal studies only, not human data, which may explain why they are only considered as guidelines rather than standards. Furthermore, the thermal effect used to establish the FCC guidelines was based on acute thermal effect. It did not even deal with chronic long-term intermittent effect. In fact, Hankin's letter also states, "exposures that comply with the FCC's guidelines generally have been presented as "safe" by many of the RF system operators and service providers who must comply with them, even though there is uncertainty about possible risk from non-thermal, intermittent exposures that may continue for years."
4. Electromagnetic fields (EMFs) can come from sources with a spectrum of frequencies. EMFs from electric power sources usually have a frequency less than 1 kHz, while radio frequency (RF) generated by SmartMeters are reportedly in the range of 900 MHz to 2.4 GHz. While overall research on the EMF health effect remains limited, there are more

reported studies examining the EMF health effect in power line frequencies (< 1 kHz) including some of my research [1–3] than in RF. It is not clear at this moment whether the findings on the EMF health effect at lower frequencies (i.e., < 1 kHz) can be applied to RF range. If the underlying mechanisms are similar, the findings in lower frequency EMFs can then be applied to RF range for SmartMeters. Many studies of power frequencies reported associations with childhood leukemia, miscarriage, poor semen quality, autoimmune diseases at a level much lower than those generating thermal damage as used by FCC.

5. Many chronic diseases that the public is concerned about (e.g., cancer) have a long latency period and take decades to show symptoms. Most wireless networks and devices have only been used widely in the last 10 to 15 years. Therefore, many studies evaluating RF health effects related to cancer risk previously, if they failed to identify an adverse health effect, are not appropriate to be used as evidence to claim the safety of RF exposure, since the latency period has not been long enough to show the effect, even if an adverse association does indeed exist.
6. While the underlying mechanisms of the potential EMF health effect are not totally understood at present, skeptics have focused on the EMF thermal effect, especially those who are NOT in the profession of biomedical research, such as physicists. It is now known that EMFs can interfere with the human body through multiple mechanisms. For example, it has been demonstrated that communication between cells depends on EMF signals, likely in a very low level. External EMFs could conceivably interfere with normal cell communication, thus disrupting normal cell differentiation and proliferation. Such disturbance could lead to miscarriage, birth defects and cancer.

To address the two questions raised in the letter:

1. Whether FCC standards for SmartMeters are sufficiently protective of public health taking into account current exposure levels to radio frequency and electromagnetic fields. First, FCC currently has only "guidelines," not standards, as explained above. Second, as described in the background information above, the current FCC guidelines only deal with thermal effect, which also was only based on animal studies. Meeting the current FCC guidelines, in the best case scenario, only means that one won't have heat damage from SmartMeter exposure. It says nothing about safety from the risk of many chronic diseases that the public is most concerned about such as cancer, miscarriage, birth defects, semen quality, autoimmune diseases, etc. Therefore, when it comes to non-thermal effects of RF, which is the most relevant effect for public concerns, FCC guidelines are irrelevant and cannot be used for any claims of SmartMeter safety unless we are addressing heat damage.
2. Whether additional technology-specific standards are needed for SmartMeter and other devices that are commonly found in and around homes to ensure adequate protection from adverse health effects. Safety standards for RF exposure related to non-thermal effects are urgently needed to protect the public from potential adverse health effects from RF exposure that are increasingly prevalent in daily life due to installation of ever-powerful wireless networks and devices like SmartMeters. Unfortunately, scientific research is still lacking in this area, and some endpoints like cancer take decades to study. The safety standards are not likely to be available anytime soon. The bottom line is that the safety level for RF exposure related to non-thermal effect is unknown at present, and whoever claims that their device

is safe regarding non-thermal effect is either ignorant or misleading.

In summary, we do not currently have scientific data to determine where the safe RF exposure level is regarding the non-thermal effects. Therefore, it should be recognized that we are dealing with uncertainty now and most likely for the foreseeable future. The question for governmental agencies, especially those concerned with public health and safety, is, given the uncertainty, should we err on the side of safety and take precautionary avoidance measures? Unknown does not mean safe.

There are two unique features regarding SmartMeter exposure. First, because of mandatory installation, it is a universal exposure. Virtually every household is exposed. Second, it is an involuntary exposure. The public that are exposed to SmartMeters do not have any input in deciding whether they would like to have the SmartMeter installed. The installation is imposed upon the public. Governmental agencies for protecting public health and safety should be much more vigilant towards involuntary environmental exposures, because governmental agencies are the only defense against such involuntary exposure. Given the uncertainty of SmartMeter safety, one rational first step of public policy could be to require household consent before installation of SmartMeters. Finally, because of the nature of universal exposure, many susceptible and vulnerable populations, including pregnant women and young children, are unknowingly exposed 24 hours a day, 7 days a week. Usually, the threshold of harm is much lower for susceptible populations.

References:

Li, D. K. et al, "A population-based prospective cohort study of personal exposure to magnetic fields during pregnancy and the risk of miscarriage," *Epidemiology*, vol. 13, no.1 (2002): 9–20.

Li, D. K. et al, "Exposure to magnetic fields and the risk of poor sperm quality," *Reproductive Toxicology*, vol. 29, no. 1 (2010): 86–92.

Li, D. K. et al, "Electric blanket use during pregnancy in relation to the risk of congenital urinary tract anomalies among women with a history of subfertility," *Epidemiology*, vol. 6, no. 5 (1995): 485–489.

American Academy of Environmental Medicine

www.aaemonline.org

January 29, 2012
On the Proposed Decision of Commissioner Peevey
Before the Public Utilities Commission of the State of California
Mailed 11/22/2011: 11-03-014

Dear Commissioners:

The Board of the American Academy of Environmental Medicine opposes the installation of wireless "smart meters" in homes and schools based on a scientific assessment of the current medical literature (references available on request). Chronic exposure to wireless radio frequency radiation is a preventable environmental hazard that is sufficiently well documented to warrant immediate preventative public health action.

As representatives of physician specialists in the field of environmental medicine, we have an obligation to urge precaution when sufficient scientific and medical evidence suggests health risks that can potentially affect large populations. The literature raises serious concern regarding the level of radio frequency (RF - 3KHz - 300 GHz) or extremely low frequency (ELF - 300 Hz) exposures produced by "smart meters" to warrant an immediate and complete moratorium on their use and deployment until further study can be performed. The Board of the American Academy of Environmental Medicine wishes to point out that existing FCC guidelines for RF safety, which have been used to justify installation of "smart meters," only look at thermal tissue damage and are obsolete, since many modern studies show metabolic and genomic damage from RF and ELF exposures below the level of intensity that heats tissue. The FCC guidelines are therefore inadequate for use in establishing public health standards. More modern literature shows medically and biologically significant effects of RF and ELF at lower energy densities. These effects accumulate over time, which is an important consideration, given the chronic nature of exposure from "smart meters." The current medical literature raises credible questions about genetic and cellular effects, hormonal effects, male fertility, blood/brain barrier damage and increased risk of certain types of cancers from RF or ELF levels similar to those emitted from "smart meters." Children are placed at particular risk for altered brain development, and impaired learning and behavior. Further, EMF/RF adds synergistic effects to the damage observed from a range of toxic chemicals.

Given the widespread, chronic, and essentially inescapable ELF/RF exposure of everyone living near a "smart meter," the Board of the American Academy of Environmental Medicine finds it unacceptable from a public health standpoint to implement this technology until these serious medical concerns are resolved. We consider a moratorium on installation of wireless "smart meters" to be an issue of the highest importance.

The Board of the American Academy of Environmental Medicine also wishes to note that the US NIEHS National Toxicology Program in 1999 cited radio frequency radiation as a potential carcinogen. Existing safety limits for pulsed RF were termed "not protective of public health" by the Radio frequency Interagency Working Group (a federal interagency working group including the FDA, FCC, OSHA, the EPA and others). Emissions given off by "smart meters" have been classified by the World Health Organization's International Agency for Research on Cancer (IARC) as a Possible Human Carcinogen.

Hence, we call for:

- An immediate moratorium on "smart meter" installation until these serious public health issues are resolved. Continuing with their installation would be extremely irresponsible.
- Modifying your revised proposed decision to include hearings on health impact in the second proceedings, along with cost evaluation and community-wide opt-out.
- Providing immediate relief to those requesting it and restoring analog meters.

Members of the Board
American Academy of Environmental Medicine

How to Prevent Deployment of Cellular Antennas and "Smart" Meters

Suggestions from Elizabeth Kelley,
public health advocate, electromagneticsafety.org

Because one cellular antenna or one transmitting utility meter affects a whole community, efforts to prevent further deployment of wireless equipment can *build* community—starting with neighbors who educate themselves about our federal laws and the health effects of exposure to radio frequency (RF) radiation.

The Telecommunications Act's Section 704 serves the industry and preempts local control. It prohibits a municipality or state from refusing a permit to install or upgrade cellular antennas based on environmental or health effects. It mandates that the FCC's guidelines for exposure to radiation are "the law of the land," and that no state can adopt lower limits to protect its citizens. Section 704 has desensitized many government agencies to peoples' valid concerns.

Still, citizens can argue successfully against new antennas by treating the equipment as a neighborhood nuisance that disturbs an area's look and/or lowers property values. To oppose cellular antenna proposals:

1. Organize a team that includes local engineers, biologists, physicians, electricians, mediators, public health workers, legislative and regulatory analysts, writers, fundraisers,

public speakers and graphic artists. Give your group a name, such as Neighbors for Safer Technology.

2. Become familiar with your state and municipal wireless telecommunications siting ordinances and how they apply to the proposal at hand.
3. If the property owner has not yet signed a lease with the wireless carrier, request a meeting with him or her to present your concerns, including health concerns. Show a film such as James Russell's "Resonance" (available at vimeo.com), Talal Jabari's "Full Signal," or "Public Exposure: DNA, Democracy and the Wireless Revolution" (available on YouTube). Keep your handout brief. If you can convince the property owner to be a good neighbor and forego the lease, the proposal will not go forward. This can happen!
4. Become familiar with the technical specifications of the proposed new antennas: their location, height, purpose (commercial, public safety/police), power level, frequencies transmitted, whether the site will be a co-location (with antennas owned by multiple carriers—i.e., AT&T, Verizon, T-Mobile). Once approved, new co-location sites are now federally regulated; no further public notice or review of upgrades will be required. Get a copy of materials submitted by the telecom carrier(s) to your town's planning department, and review them.
5. Make sure that all technical and local code requirements are met. For example, historic neighborhoods often have special requirements. Monitor the application's progress for any developments by keeping in touch with your planning department.
6. If a lease has been signed, evaluate the permit application that the wireless carrier(s) submitted to your planning and land use department. Visit the proposed site with engineers and contractors who know local code requirements. List issues

to raise in the zoning hearing. (Will height requirements be violated? Will a cell tower made to look like a palm tree disrupt the neighborhood's character?) Stay in touch with your planning and land use staff to keep abreast of the review schedule, hearing dates, and changes to the application.

7. Keep your neighbors informed. Make a flyer that describes the proposal. Hold educational forums. You might feature a film or an expert speaker and give attendees a chance to voice their questions and concerns. Write a petition that briefly outlines your neighborhood's concerns. While the permit review process cannot take your health concerns into account, you are not precluded from expressing health concerns in your petition. Actually, going door-to-door to share your concerns, especially within the proposed antenna site's first 300 to 500 feet, is very important. Explain that permits have been denied in other parts of the country when residents argue that viewing a cell tower—whether it is disguised or not—from inside a home will adversely affect the view, the neighborhood's character and subsequently devalue property. Noise (from the HVAC and generators that support an installation and from increased traffic caused by maintenance workers) will also disrupt the neighborhood, impact its character and lower property values. FHA financing and commercial mortgage refinancing will become more difficult. Set up a table at your farmers' market. Submit editorials to local papers. Brief public officials one-on-one. Get informed, level-headed speakers interviewed on local radio shows and by print reporters.
8. Typically, the wireless carrier(s) that propose a new antenna will be required to hold neighborhood meetings to describe their proposal and answer questions. This is a chance to inform everyone who attends about the health risks of the proposed antenna and to ask the carriers' reps detailed

questions about the proposal. If the reps or planning and land use staff say that attendees cannot talk about health at the meeting, clarify that the First Amendment allows us to speak freely. The federal preemption that prevents consideration of health concerns applies only to the formal hearing process when the government agency reviews and decides whether to approve or deny a permit application.

9. Whether public officials deny or grant a permit for an antenna, they are concerned about their community's health. Ask them to pass a resolution that acknowledges their concerns about the health effects of RF electromagnetic radiation and about federal preemptions that can prevent them from denying cellular antenna permit applications. The resolution could call for repeal of the TCA's Section 704, restoration of local control over the siting and management of commercial antennas, lowering the FCC's current RF exposure limits and/or recognition that biological creatures are affected by radiation emitted by wireless devices and telecom equipment. Pima County, Arizona, Los Angeles County, California and Marin County, California and other local governments have passed such resolutions. See CloutNow.org for more info.
10. At the hearings, show your political will! Ask people to attend and testify, to provide information specific to the proposed site that could lead to a denial of the permit application. Show pictures to illustrate the tower's visual impact on the neighborhood as well as the radiation pattern that will be imposed on existing homes, schools and health care facilities within a mile radius. Enlarge graphics found at antennasearch.com to show the antennas and towers already located within a four-mile radius of the proposed site.
11. For more info, see Cell Tower Safety: A Citizen's Tool Box, at emrpolicy.org/public_policy/siting_zoning/index.htm.

Smart Meters

Preventing further deployment of "smart" meters requires different tactics. Since 2005, following enactment of the Federal Energy Policy Act and initial funding under the American Recovery and Reinvestment Act of 2009, the U.S. Department of Energy's Smart Grid Program has provided annual demonstration grants to spur "innovation" and expedite deployment. State public utility commissions have promoted "smart" metering, supposedly to achieve efficiency and conservation. While utility companies and public utility commissions are not prohibited from considering concerns about "smart" meters, they have worked hard to overcome customer objections, including those based on meters' effects on health, privacy, fire hazards, the grid's susceptibility to hacking and higher customer utility bills.

Many cities and counties have implemented moratoriums on "smart" meters' installation in order to allow time to study concerns about health, privacy and cost-effectiveness. While a moratorium is not binding and may not impede a utility company's activities, it sends a strong political message to state utility regulators and state legislators. California, Maine and Vermont have conducted health studies. Maine conducted a cost-effectiveness study. Several administrative appeals and lawsuits have been filed at the state level and in federal courts. Some states have contested the overall cost-effectiveness of the "smart" Grid. Some utilities have created opt-out or self-reading programs for ratepayers who prefer to keep their analog meters.

Meanwhile, the race is on to complete installation of the program across the country. Unfortunately, the burden of proof that transmitting meters harm, as well as the burden of refusing a transmitting digital "smart" meter and insisting on a mechanical meter, fall on citizen-ratepayers.

Here are some suggestions for utility customers and local government agencies to get their concerns addressed:

1. Ask your local government to pass a moratorium on installing any "smart" meters to permit a "study period" that studies "smart" meters' health effects, cost/benefits, fire safety, privacy issues and erroneous billing issues. Many communities in California and British Columbia have adopted such moratoriums. Stopsmartmeters.org has more info.
2. Write down the make and model numbers of each meter (for electric, gas and water) on your property, and learn as much as you can about them. Do any transmit radiofrequencies? If so, how often? You may have to rent or borrow an RF meter to determine each meter's duty cycle. Utilities may under-report the duty cycle. *Some "smart" meters emit microbursts 15,000 times each day.* Research your utility companies' schedules for updating their meters. Learn about their self-reading programs and opt-out plans.
3. Do any of the meters on your property interfere with your TV, medical implants, sleep apnea machines or other appliances or devices? Find out if/when transmitting meters were placed on your property. Has anyone's health in your household changed since then? Pay particular attention to health or behavioral changes in children and pets.
4. Secure your analog meter with a lock so that it can't be removed.
5. Send the utility a certified letter that refuses the installation of an RF transmitting meter on your property and that requests placement on their permanent opt-out list (see Jerry Day's suggested letter in the appendices).
6. Require utility workers who enter your property to show company identification. If the utility company contacts you

about installing a new meter, ask for the make and model number *before installers arrive* and research it. Tell installers that you do not permit them to enter property or to install a new meter without your permission; and, if you prefer, without your being present. If they trespass your property, call police. Form a neighborhood watch. Film encounters with utility meter installers. *If you or your neighbors already have an RF transmitting meter installed*:

7. Keep your distance from it (pets, children and plants, too) as well as you can. With varying success, some people have shielded the meters. Seek advice from a qualified electrical engineer to ensure that shielding is properly installed. Recognize that "smart" meters on neighboring homes and businesses may increase RF emission levels around your home that you cannot control.
8. With a certified letter (a sample is available at freedomtaker.com), revoke your consent to have the transmitting meter installed and set a deadline for its removal. Insist that the replacement meter be an electromechanical analog meter. Request that the utility confirm that its replacement (to an electro-mechanical analog meter) be in writing.

Don't be a NIMBY. Advocate for needed changes in federal policies that will ensure more health protections and restore local control over public utilities (electricity, gas, water and telecommunications) that provide essential services to benefit society. Once you've gained experience in opposing antennas or "smart" meters, pay it forward by sharing with others what you have learned.

How to Refuse a Residential Radiation-Emitting Surveillance Meter

A Model Letter Offered by www.jerryday.com

Jerry Day posts the following letter for anyone who chooses to refuse installation of a "smart" meter on their residence or property. He suggests that you consult your attorney to tailor the letter to your specifications, then send your revised version to your utility company's CEO or president by certified mail.

Keep copies of your letter and your certified mail receipt.

If anyone attempts to install a transmitting meter on your residence, show them the copy of your letter and proof of its delivery (your certified mail receipt). Tell them that installing a transmitting meter on your residence will thereby be a criminal trespass. If they attempt this, you will call the police, request that the installer be taken into custody, and file a criminal complaint with the police.

If the company responds to your letter in writing, Jerry Day suggests that you write back. Remind them that they have not proven that they may lawfully install any radiation-emitting surveillance device on your residence.

Model Letter

Your Name/Energy Customer's Name
Street Address
City, State Zip Code

Utility's CEO, President, General Manager, or Board Chair
Utility Company
Street Address
City, State Zip Code

Date

NOTICE OF NO CONSENT TO TRESPASS, SURVEILLANCE OR RADIATION POLLUTION. NOTICE OF LIABILITY. ADHESION CONTRACT.

Dear (CEO's Name) and All Agents, Officers, Employees, Contractors and Interested Parties:

In regard to your possible intention to install a "smart" or other digital utility meter at the above address, those meters violate the law. They cause endangerment to people in their vicinity owing to the following factors:

1. They individually identify electrical devices and record when they are operated, causing invasion of privacy.
2. They monitor household activity and occupancy in violation of rights and domestic privacy.
3. They transmit wireless signals that are interceptable by unauthorized and distant parties.
4. No power company or other individual agency has consent to conduct surveillance or monitoring or to emit radiation (EMR) on our property or residence with a digital meter.
5. Those with access to the data can review a permanent history of household activities taken and viewed unlawfully

and without the consent of occupants and subjects of the surveillance.

6. Those databases may be shared with, or fall into the hands of, unauthorized law enforcement, private hackers of wireless transmissions and other unidentified parties for use against the interests of the energy subscribers and the occupants of the structures.
7. "Smart" meters are, by definition, surveillance devices that violate federal and state wiretapping laws by recording and storing databases of private and personal activities and behaviors recorded without the consent or knowledge of those people who are monitored.
8. It is possible, for example, with analysis of certain "smart" meter data, for unauthorized and distant parties to determine medical conditions, sexual activities, vacancy patterns, general affluence, trade secrets and physical locations of occupants.
9. By intentional transmission and/or incidental disruption of house current, digital meters emit cancer-causing electromagnetic radiation, which violates laws against public endangerment, assault and commission of bodily harm.
10. Digital meters are designed to transmit using electromagnetic radiation known to cause cancer and many other diseases, illnesses and symptoms.

For these reasons, and by right of occupancy and property ownership, I prohibit, and deny consent of, any installation and use of any monitoring, eavesdropping, surveillance and radiation emitting devices on my property and place of residence, especially in the form of a digital, transmitting utility meter.

Any attempt to install any such device directed at me or other occupants on my property or place of residence will constitute trespass, stalking, wiretapping and assault, all prohibited and punishable by law through criminal and civil actions.

All persons, government agencies and private organizations responsible for installing or operating monitoring devices that I consider unlawful will be fully liable for major financial and compliance claims and demands in excess of one million dollars.

This is legal notice. The liabilities and obligations listed above are true and binding upon all parties upon delivery of this notice. These terms and conditions apply without regard to status or existence of any "opt-out" contract.

Under my authority as owner and/or occupant of the above property, and under your implied or expressed application to enter that property, this is an adhesion contract to which you are now bound until and unless you respond with factual rebuttal in a sworn statement by an authorized and identified party within 21 days of this delivery. Any rebuttal must show your authority to install an unlawful radiation-emitting surveillance device (digital electric "meter") on my property without my consent. Expect rebuttal to any such claim. Any failure to timely show and prove full and binding authority to install the unlawful and harmful device on my property and/or place of occupancy will be an agreement with all terms and conditions herein. I/we deny and refuse any past, present and future proposal, offer, demand or claim contrary to any terms or conditions herein.

Notice to principle is notice to agent, and notice to agent is notice to principal.

Signature

Name of energy user and/or customer

Note: If a utility company has already installed a transmitting meter on your residence and you want it removed, first find out if the company allows an opt-out. If they do, simply go through the proper channels for having it removed and replaced with a mechanical meter. If opt-outs are not available in your area, Jerry Day offers a letter that demands removal at www.freedomtaker.com.

How to Detect EMFs

For a crude way to measure the presence of EMFs, get a $15 portable *analog* radio (model 12-467 or 12-586 from Radio Shack).

Turn the radio to AM. Tune it away from clearly heard stations. "White noise" is the sound of lightning, the sun's emissions and very low human-made frequencies. This static is not considered a problem. A hard-edged buzz—most prominent near things with lots of power such as refrigerators, laundry dryers, monitors, printers and dimmer switches—signals electrical or magnetic fields.

Hold the radio parallel to the floor, near outlets and cords. If the radio buzzes, then you've detected an electrical or magnetic field. Try the same thing holding the radio perpendicular to the floor.

If you turn off your main breaker and still hear a buzz, then the problem's source is *outside* of your house, perhaps with a neighbor and/or with the power lines or your neighborhood transformer.

If you turn off your main breaker and the buzz stops, then the problem is *within* your house. In this case, turn the main breaker back on and turn individual breakers off one at a time to see which one is the source of the problem.

Once you've collected information, you'll need an electrician and/or a utility company technician who'll respect your research, help you identify the specific source(s) of EMFs—and correct errors. Note that while most electromagnetic fields can be reduced, most electricians are not trained to respond to a buzz as a biological hazard.

Karl Riley's book, *Tracing EMFs in Building Wiring and Grounding*, Edward Leeper's *Silencing the Fields: A Practical Guide to Reducing AC Magnetic Fields*, and Marv Loftness' *AC Powerline Interference Handbook* (which describes problems on the utility side) are all excellent guides.

A $7 circuit tester with a three-pronged plug and three lights will tell you if the ground, hot and neutral are correctly wired at each outlet.

Also note that a radio may not pick up problems caused by wireless devices, since they operate in the microwave range, and AM radio does not operate in those frequencies. That said, near a cell phone or a laptop, your AM radio might hiss to signal a higher frequency field.

For a more accurate reading, rent a magnometer or a spectrum analyzer; www.magneticsciences.com has an excellent Q&A section about measuring magnetic fields and RFs from various sources—and the kinds of meters that can detect different sources. Magnetic Sciences also rents and sells different kinds of meters for measuring different sources of radiation.

A Timeline of Electronic Developments

With the introduction of each new technology, ambient levels of radiation increase.

Telephones

1844 First news dispatched by electric telegraph invented by Samuel Morse. "What hath God wrought?" Morse asked, in his first communication.

1876 First complete sentence transmitted via telephone invented by Alexander Graham Bell.

1879 First telephone exchange outside of the U.S., in London, England.

1883 First telephone exchange linking two cities: New York and Boston.

Electricity

1878 First successful demonstration of incandescent lightbulb by Joseph Swan.

1879 Thomas Edison presents the first commercially viable incandescent lightbulb. The first street lighting is installed in Cleveland, Ohio.

1882 First electric power plant station in New York City, designed by Thomas Edison.

1890 Edison's studies of the dangers of electrocution from alternating current electricity lead to the electric chair, a device that could put condemned criminals to death.

1901 First power line opened between Canada and the U.S.

1908 Electric vacuum cleaners and washing machines go on the market.

Broadcasting

1896 First wireless transmission over 30 km. by Nikola Tesla.
1900 First audio radio transmission by Reginald Fessenden.
1902 First transatlantic radio wave transmission by Guglielmo Marconi.
1906 Amplitude modulation radio (AM) invented by Reginald Fesseden.
1922 Broadcasting "boom" in the U.S.
1933 Frequency modulation radio (FM) invented by Edwin Howard Armstrong.

Radar

1904 First demonstration of the use of radio echoes for detecting ships with a Remote Object Viewing Device (*Telemobiloskop*), by Christian Hülsmeyer.
1937 World's first operative radar network in the UK, called Chain Home.
1945 Microwave oven invented by Percy Spencer.
1948 Radar is introduced for traffic law enforcement.
1967 First home microwave oven is sold by Amana in the U.S.

Television

1926 First demonstration of a working television by Baird, in the UK.
1927 First televised speech transmitted from Washington, DC, to New York.
1928 First color television demonstrated by John Logie Baird.
1941 Commercial TV service becomes available in the U.S.
1952 First TV broadcast in Canada.

Computers

1941 First operational computer by Konrad Zuse (the Z machine).

1951 First commercially produced computer, UNIVAC I (Universal Automatic Computer).
1953 IBM releases its first mass-produced electronic computer, IBM 701.
1981 IBM introduces its personal computer (PC), IBM 5150.
1982 *Time Magazine* names the personal computer "Machine of the Year."
1984 Apple Computer launches the first successful mouse-driven computer.
1993 IBM releases the first commercial portable computer, the ThinkPad.

Mobile Phones

1956 First fully automatic mobile phone system installed in Sweden by TeliaSonera and Ericsson.
1971 Zero Generation: the first truly successful public mobile phone network, in Finland.
1980 First Generation: analog mobile phone networks (NMT, APS).
1983 First handheld mobile phones become commercially available in the U.S.
1984 First cordless phones introduced (CTI).
1990 2nd Generation (2G): Digital mobile phone networks (GSM, TDMA, CDMA).
1991 Digitally enhanced cordless (DECT) phones become available.
2000 3rd Generation (3G): Digital mobile phone networks installed (CDMA 2000, WCDDMA, UMTS, HSPA, HSPA).
2010 4th Generation (4G): digital mobile phone networks installed (LTE-Advanced, WirelessMAN-Advanced; pre-4G; LTE; WiMax).

Computer Networks

1965 Two computers communicate with each other for the first time.

1969 Based on packet-switching technology, a two-letter message is sent via Arpanet from a computer at UCLA to another at Stanford University.

1970 First wireless computer communication network installed, at the University of Hawaii (Alohanet).

1972 E-mail is introduced.

1973 First trans-Atlantic connection via Arpanet, from the Information Sciences Institute in California to the University College of London.

1973 First wired Ethernet network connects the first laser printer to more than 100 computers at Xerox.

1985 First domain name registered: Symbolics.com.

1991 In Switzerland, CERN launches the World Wide Web.

1993 CERN announces that anyone can use the World Wide Web for free.

1999 First wireless LAN or Wi-Fi becomes available to home users (AirPort).

2004 Jerusalem becomes the world's first city to offer free Wi-Fi.

Convergence of Communication Devices

1992 Designed by IBM, the first smartphone includes a calendar, an address book, a world clock, a calculator, games, and the ability to email and fax.

1996 First Web browser for a mobile phone (Apple Newton) is introduced.

1997 First pictures made with a smartphone and shared instantly over the Internet.

2001 First "smart" electricity grid deployed in Italy.

2006 Cloud computing offered to external customers by Amazon Web Services.

2009 The first "smart" appliance (a hot water tank).

Glossary of Terms

4G Service for "fourth generation" wireless devices, including smart phones.

alternating current (AC) An electric field that reverses direction at a given frequency along with the current and the voltage that creates the field. AC is associated with an oscillating frequency or vibration. Our utility companies provide electricity through AC, usually 50 or 60 Hz.

ampere A unit of measure of current or charge flow.

antenna An electrical structure that transmits or receives electromagnetic waves. The efficiency of an antenna is a function of its size, shape, and geometry, as well as the frequency and polarization (orientation) of the EM wave. Corroding metal dental material in one's mouth may act as a complete radio receiver with an inefficient antenna.

arcing An electrical spark—like a little lightning bolt—that occurs when the air of another insulator breaks down between conductors.

bandwidth The range of frequencies used to transmit data, whether or not the data is sent within cables or by a wireless device. Video requires more bandwidth than voice; voice requires more bandwidth than text.

battery A device that stores electrical energy through chemical reactions.

The BioInitiative 2012 Report 1800 studies linking health impacts such as DNA damage, brain tumors, childhood cancers, auto-immune diseases, breast cancer, and Alzheimer's to electromagnetic fields and wireless technologies. www.bioinitiative.org.

broadband An Internet connection with high bandwidth (a large range of frequencies) that allows large amounts of data for a movie or video game, for example, to be transmitted quickly.

broadband over power lines (BPL) High-speed Internet access on existing electrical wires, rather than on phone wires or Ethernet wires.

capacitor Also called a "condenser" or a "Leyden Jar," a device that stores energy by charge separation on conductors separated by an insulator.

carrier frequency The base frequency of a transmitter to which both the transmitter and the receiver are tuned to communicate—i.e., for TV, radio, mobile phones, or wireless Internet to function.

cellular phone A phone that operates without wires within a *cell.* A cell is an area of about .8 miles, created by a base station (a cellular antenna). In a moving car, a cell phone transfers from one antenna to the next about every .8 miles.

charge A fundamental property of certain particles that creates an electrical field, notably the electron and proton. Usually, electrons are more important than protons, because electrons are smaller and can move faster.

conduction The response of electrons to the application of an electric field inside a material. Many electrons moving as a current generate heat by collisions and scattering (momentum transfer).

conductor Material that allows relatively free motion of electrons.

corded landline phone A phone that plugs into a wall-jack; the handset (mouthpiece or microphone and earpiece or speaker) connects to the base by a cord.

cordless landline phone A phone that plugs into a wall-jack but has no cord between the handset and the base. Communication between the base and the handset occurs wirelessly, by microwave radio signals. Older cordless phones used simple radio modulation that was easily eavesdropped. Newer models use frequency hopping and/or digital encryption to improve privacy.

current Movement or flow of charge, measured in amperes.

digital electronics use electric pulses turned on and off quickly to send information between two locations or to process and store information. The quick on-and-off creates harmonics, and the sequence of pulses creates modulation, neither of which occur in nature.

direct current (DC) Electric current that moves in one direction only, such as current produced by a battery.

dirty power (also called dirty electricity) If clean electricity (which some say does not exist, in practice) is a perfectly smooth AC wave at 60 Hz, high frequencies or pulses on the wires can chop up current and disrupt power quality. RF pulses, for example, operate at much higher frequencies than the usual harmonics. Although engineers have long recognized dirty power can damage electronics and waste energy, few have recognized dirty power's effects on health.

electrical field A basic property of a charged particle, most commonly the electron. An electric field creates a force that causes other charges to move. Moving charges are called a current. The strength and direction of the forces that would be exerted on a charge within the electrical field is determined by voltage between charges a distance apart. An electrical field is measured in volts per meter.

electric grid Infrastructure that generates and delivers electricity from power generating stations to substations, neighborhood transformers, homes, schools, hospitals, and businesses—and back to the generating stations.

electrical transient noise In an electrical circuit, temporary bursts of voltage or charge that interrupt their intended signal.

This electrical interference can often be heard as a hum, a buzz, or crackling on a radio.

electrocution An electric shock of about 100 milliamperes across the heart producing death. Higher currents may also cause burns.

electromagnetic compatibility (EMC) measures the ability of two electrical or electromagnetic devices to perform their correct function without causing interference to each other.

electromagnetic field Although this can include electric fields, magnetic fields, or both at once, an electric field does not always create a flow of charge. When it does, this flow of charge or current generates a magnetic field.

electromagnetic interference (EMI) occurs when one device prevents another device from operating or performing correctly. EMI may typically occur by conduction (direct electrical contact), induction (nearby time-changing magnetic field), electromagnetic radiation, or, less commonly, in capacitive coupling.

electromagnetic radiation (EMR) refers to electromagnetic waves that carry energy from their source at the speed of light. It occurs when charged particles change their velocity by acceleration or deceleration.

electron A fundamental particle in the Standard Particle Model that physicists use to describe the universe around us. Electrons are responsible for about 90% of the processes in our daily experience.

EMF can stand for electromagnetic field or electro-motive force.

Environmental Protection Agency (EPA) The federal agency that regulates non-thermal ionizing radiation in the environment from natural or artificial sources. Currently, EPA activities related to RF safety and health are advisory; epa.gov/radtown/basic.html See also NIOSH.

Federal Communications Commission (FCC) The federal agency that regulates radio frequency transmitters to prevent interference to communication in non-federal governments (i.e., states, and municipalities). Federal transmitters are coordinated by the National Telecommunications Information Administration. FCC.gov; NTIA.doc.gov.

Federal Drug Administration Center for Devices and Radiological Health, FDA CDRH is concerned with the health effects of exposure to color TVs, microwave ovens, and mobile phones as well as medical devices, www.cdrh.fda.gov; cdc.gov; osha.gov/SLTC/radio frequencyradiation/index.html.

ferrite Magnetic insulator that is used in transformers and to suppress RFs traveling along wires.

fiber optics Very thin, transparent cables that carry signals by pulsing light. Fiber optic cables offer the fastest connection, the greatest capacity, the most security, and the lowest EMR of available technology. They require much less electrical power than antennas to transmit signals.

filter A device that removes some frequency fields of electromagnetic energy.

frequency The number of times per second that either the electric or the magnetic field completes a full cycle (a positive extreme falling to a negative extreme and increasing back to the positive extreme). Measured in cycles-per-second (CPS) or hertz.

gauss A unit of magnetic field. It measures intensity (strength and direction) of a magnetic field through a surface. Note: In standardized units, gauss has been replaced by "tesla." One tesla = 10,000 gauss. 10G = 1 milliT = 0.001 T. The Earth's magnetic field at DC is roughly 50,000 nanotesla or 0.05 millitesla.

gigahertz (GHz) One billion cycles per second.

ground There are two main kinds of ground. An *earth ground* is a connection to a ground rod buried in the dirt. Found at a house's circuit panel and at utility poles and transformers, the earth ground connection is intended to keep the voltage of a conductor close to zero. Every outlet has a *safety ground,* which only carries current in the event of a fault. Normally, the safety ground carries no current (excepting a tiny current from capacitive coupling). Ground current fault interrupters (GCFIs) are designed to detect excessive ground currents and interrupt (like a circuit breaker) the current to protect people and animals from electrocution.

harmonics Integer (or whole number 1, 2, 3...) multiples of the base frequency. For example, if 60 Hz is the base frequency, the harmonics would be at 120 Hz, 180 Hz, and so on.

hertz (Hz) The unit of measurement of frequency—like a pound is a measurement of weight. Hertz is the number of cycles or vibrations completed in one second. Hertz can refer to anything that changes in time—like ocean waves, sound waves, or electromagnetic fields. See *frequency*.

induction The use of a rapidly changing magnetic field in order to cause a current to flow in a good conductor (some stove-top ovens cause heating in metal pans this way).

inductor A device that stores electrical energy in a magnetic field.

insulator Material that impedes or resists motion of most electrons.

ionizing The production of ions from neutral atoms by exposure to radiation with sufficient strength to dislodge an electron using a single photon. X-ray machines and nuclear power plants emit ionizing radiation, as do some natural materials called isotopes—such as uranium, thorium, radium, and radon. The dislodged electron is called an ion.

kilohertz (kHz) One thousand vibrations per second.

magnetic field A magnetic field is created by a moving charged particle or current. A time-varying magnetic field creates a force that also causes charges to move. Measured in units called gauss (G) or tesla (T), the BioInitiative Report recommends limiting magnetic fields to 1.0 mG or 0.1 mT. OSHA allows workers exposure up to 1000 mG. No agency regulates exposure for the general public. Studies show that exposure to magnetic fields above 2.5 mG causes increases in childhood leukemia. At close range, a typical electric alarm clock generates between 10 and 30 mG.

megahertz (MHz) One million cycles per second.

microwave A kind of radio frequency field. An electromagnetic field with frequency between 300 MHz and 300 GHz. Also used to describe a microwave oven that heats food by causing rapid rotation of the water molecule in response to a rapidly changing RF field at 2.4 GHz.

milligauss (mG) One thousandth of one gauss.

modulation The method of imposing information on a transmitted carrier frequency. There are many different ways to accomplish this. A few examples are:

amplitude modulations Amplitude variations in the carrier wave without changing the carrier frequency. Used for AM radio.

frequency modulations Modulation used by FM radio.

OAM Used for cable TV.

non-ionizing radiation The part of the electromagnetic spectrum that extends from zero frequency (DC) to the frequencies of visible light. It does not contain sufficient intrinsic energy to cause ionization of atoms in the body's chemicals. RF radiation is non-ionizing, because it is not capable of "ionizing" an atom using a single photon, and can only ignite atoms using multiple photons when the field is very strong, as in a fluorescent light or a lightning bolt.

OSHA Occupational Safety and Health Administration; OSHA .gov; regulates workers' safety and health.

phase AC electricity is sometimes phased, which shifts it in time to keep the return wire running the same amount of current all the time. If you hold your elbows tight to your side and bring both hands up and then down to together, they are moving *in phase* (or zero degrees phase angle). Raise your left hand while lowering your right hand, then raise your right while lowering your left, and your hands are *out-of-phase* (90 degrees phase angle). More complicated motions are possible and used to efficiently control certain kinds of motors. The phase is also the difference in arrival time for an acoustic signal arriving at your ears that allows you to locate someone talking to you.

The Precautionary Principle Similar to the Hippocratic oath, "First, do no harm," the Precautionary Principle suggests that we not use a technology or product when its safety is unknown and alternatives are available. Scientists, farmers, and breast-cancer action groups developed the Precautionary Principle in 1998 after observing that many consumers assume that products such as pesticides are safe just because they are in the marketplace. But these products actually harm health when used repeatedly or in combination with other hazardous products.

radiation Energy that travels through space or through matter. In telecommunications, the frequency of electromagnetic radiation in part determines the extent to which it can carry data and can penetrate metal roofs, thick walls, and people. See *ionizing* and *non-ionizing radiation.*

radio-frequency (RF) Electromagnetic radiation at frequencies between 30 kHz and 300 GHz.

satellite Stationed in space, telecom satellites transmit information to Earth by microwave radiation. This technology allows data to be distributed to remote locations, including places blocked by mountains or an ocean. It is used by nationally-distributed TV networks, phone providers, the military, and newspapers. Satellite dishes used on homes for satellite TV use active electronics to convert the signals to lower frequencies that can then be sent to your TV using standard coax cables. These conversion devices are another source of radiation and high-frequency transients.

Specific Absorption Rate (SAR) Exposure of tissue to EMR is measured by SAR, the ratio of power to weight (Watt/kilogram) at a given frequency above 100 kHz for a given period of time. In its regulation of mobile phones, the FCC allows a SAR of 1.6 W/kg averaged over any 1 gram of tissue. Exceptions are the extremities of the body (hands, wrists, feet, ankles and outer ear parts), where the peak spatial-average SAR limit is 4.0 W/kg averaged over any 10 grams of tissue. Exposures may be averaged over a time period not to exceed 30 minutes. Note: SAR is an EMR dosage measurement, but the FCC's SAR limit does not account for differences in exposure experienced by fetuses, infants, children, and adults or people with medical implants, nor for exposure to multiple transmitters at the same time. Some medical implant manufacturers recommended exposure limits of no more than 0.25 W/kg for fifteen minutes (www.MRIsafety.com).

second-hand SAR (like second-hand smoke) occurs from exposure to EMR sources without benefit. Second-hand SAR occurs from being near another person using a mobile phone or Wi-Fi. The FCC provides no regulation of second-hand SAR.

switch-mode power supply (SMPS) See definition for *transformer*.

tesla A unit of magnetic field; 1 tesla = 10,000 gauss (see *gauss*).

thermal effect Inductive or radiative heating of biological tissue beyond the tissue's ability to cool itself through blood flow or sweat, resulting in damage and death to the tissue.

transformer A device that changes electrical voltage and current using induction and magnetic fields. Also, a device that reduces RF energy by low pass filtering. A transformer can be the size of a city block or as small as a "wall wart" at the end of a cell phone battery charger. At close range, transformers always create magnetic fields. Newer transformers for electronics (switch mode power supplies) are smaller and more energy efficient, but they create square waves with harmonics that go to the many MHzs. The strongest electric and magnetic fields often come from the switching power supply.

transient An event that is short in duration compared to its repetition rate. A volcanic eruption can be called a transient phenomenon; so can a lightning bolt or an earthquake. A transient can occur from turning on a light switch. A transient can produce heat, sound, light, or an electromagnetic field.

voltage The measure of the amount of energy required to move a charge between two points. Voltage is potential energy. An electric field is voltage over distance (V/m). With water pressure in a pipe, until a valve is opened, no water flows. Similarly, in an electrical circuit, no electrical current (charge) flows until the circuit is completed by turning a switch on.

wavelength The distance an electromagnetic wave travels in one cycle. High frequencies have shorter wavelengths than low frequencies. Lower frequency (longer wavelength) EM waves penetrate materials better up to light frequencies. At low frequencies, the ability of a passing EM wave to make charged particles move and absorb energy is more important in determining depth of penetration. (Compared to atomic spacing, wavelengths are long.) At x-ray and gamma-ray frequencies, the wavelengths are so much shorter than atomic spacing that they behave more like particles than waves, and the density of scattering atoms becomes more important than electrical or magnetic material properties (which describe the ability of charge to move in a material.) Scattering and density are like the ability to shoot a marble (x-ray) across a table covered densely with billiard balls (atoms): the more balls are on the table, the less likely the marble can cross the table.

Wi-Fi lets people with mobile devices access the Internet wirelessly. Wi-Fi operates at 2.4 GHz, a frequency that is regulated by the FCC—while the FDA regulates microwave ovens, which operate at 2.45 GHz.

WiMax Worldwide Interoperability for Microwave Access. A wireless system that transmits broadband signals up to 30 miles from an antenna. WiMax provides wireless Internet access with a significantly stronger signal than Wi-Fi.

wireless devices Cordless DECT phones, mobile phones, iPads, "smart" digital transmitting utility meters, digital cameras, modern cars, baby monitors, doorbells, remote-controlled toys, GPS networks, alarm systems, and Wi-Fi that work without cables. Most TV remote controls use infra-red, which does not pose the same health risks as microwave wireless devices, since infrared wavelengths cannot penetrate deeper than skin.

x-ray Penetrating electromagnetic radiation that takes a picture through the skin's surface to image a bone, for example. Some airport body scanners use pulsed microwaves to operate, and some use X-rays. X-rays use such high frequencies that electrically conductive materials can't block them; only heavy nuclei like lead can (see *wavelength*).

Glossary of Acronyms

AAP	American Academy of Pediatrics
AC	alternating current
ADA	Americans with Disabilities Act
ADHD	Attention Deficit Hyperactive Disorder
AFCI	arc fault circuit interrupter
A/m	amperes per meter
AM	amplitude modulated
AMI	advanced metering infrastructure
AMR	automated meter reading
ASC	autism spectrum conditions
BPL	broadband over power lines
CFL	compact fluorescent light
CTIA	Cellular Telephone and Internet Association
DAS	distributed antenna system
DBS	deep brain stimulator
DC	direct current
DECT	digital enhanced cordless telecommunications
DOJ	Department of Justice
EHS	electro-hypersensitivity syndrome
EIS	environmental impact study
ELF	extremely low frequency
EMF	electromagnetic fields
EMR	electromagnetic radiation
EMRPI	Electromagnetic Radiation Policy Institute
FCC	Federal Communications Commission
FDA	Food and Drug Administration
FM	frequency modulated
GAO	Government Accountability Office
GBM	glioblastoma multiforme (brain cancer)

GFCI	ground fault circuit interrupter
GHz	gigahertz
GPS	Global Positioning System
GSM	Global System for Mobile Communications
GWEN	Ground Wave Emergency Network
HPWREN	High Performance Wireless Research and Educational Network
Hz	hertz
IARC	International Agency for Research on Cancer
IEEE	Institute of Electrical and Electronics Engineers
kV	kilovolts
MBTA	Migratory Bird Treaty Act
mG	milligauss
MHz	megahertz
MRI	magnetic resonance imaging
NAS	National Academies of Science
NEC	National Electric Code
NEPA	National Environmental Policy Act
NESC	National Electrical Safety Code
NFPA	National Fire Protection Association
NIOSH	National Institute for Occupational Safety and Health
NTIA	National Telecommunications and Information Agency
NTP	National Toxicology Program
PG&E	Pacific Gas and Electric
RF	radio frequency
RFIAW	Radio Frequency Interagency Work Group
SDSU	San Diego State University
SMPS	switch-mode power supply
T	tesla
TCA	Telecommunications Act of 1996
USFWS	United States Fish and Wildlife Service

UHF	ultra high frequencies
μT	microtesla
VDT	video display terminal
VHF	very high frequencies
WHO	World Health Organization
W/kg	watts per kilogram

Index

Acknowledgements

This book's substance comes from its contributors. Each of them has my profound gratitude for sharing their experience and insight from living in an electrified world.

Dr. Gary Olhoeft taught me about electricity, electronics, wireless technologies, and regulatory issues with great patience and clarity. He included physics, electrical engineering, biology, chemistry, regulations, and kitchen-table thinking in our tutorials—and never wavered from wanting *everyone* more informed. Thank you, Gary. I also thanks Kathy Sander for her delightful welcome of my very frequent calls to their household.

Janet Newton, president of the EMR Policy Institute, gave me her steady memory, dedication, insights, and encouragement. Many a day, Janet connected dots and kept me going.

Without the *BioInitiative Reports*, the Herculean work of Cindy Sage, MA and David Carpenter, MD, studies about the health and environmental effects of EMFs and EMR would be much less accessible. Their work makes books like this one possible.

Ginger Farver's courage and commitment to inform mothers about the dangers of EMR from wireless devices have touched this book more than I can say.

Bill Bruno, PhD, Paul Elliot, Brad Holian, PhD, Sonia Hoglander, Catherine Kleiber, Bruce McCreary, Whitney Seymour, Jr., David Stupin, PhD, Frank Clegg, and anonymous others reviewed early drafts of key chapters and gave edits that made the book significantly clearer.

Dr. Tom Hsu's *Integrative Science: An Investigative Approach,* Mike Holt's *Illustrated Guide to Electrical Theory* and Karl Riley's *Tracing EMFs in Building Grounding and Wiring Errors* allowed me to read (and reread) about electricity.

Albert Robinson, medical librarian extraordinaire, managed to get me a copy of Jaakko Malmivuo and Robert Plonsey's wonderful book, *Bioelectromagnetism.*

Nina Beety, Deb Carney, Sandy Fields, Larry Glover, Suzan Harjo, Michele Hertz, Libby Kelley, Catherine Kleiber, Lindsay Martell, Sandi Maurer, Susan Roberson, Michael Schwaebe and Char Zehfus each directed me to documents or people with critical information or stories.

Michael Darter and Heidi Volpe, my landlords, rode the learning curve with me with intelligence and grace while we discovered and remedied one house's quirky wiring errors.

Kay Carlson's computer help—and her encouragement—made this book possible. Jayne Cotten and Diane Jennings showed up with good cheer when Kay could not.

Throughout the ages (and more so in digital times), publishing has primarily been an educational venture, rarely a commercial one. Generous, much appreciated donations from several anonymous donors, Lisa Bloom, Christie Dodson, the Flow Fund Circle, the Life Link, the New Hampshire Charitable Foundation and Kate's Fund for Women at the Santa Fe Community Foundation supported me while I wrote. My heartfelt thanks to each of them for their belief in this project.

My hat goes off to jacket designer Kendra Arnold, who somehow took a web of complex issues and made an inviting, simple picture.

Christie Dodson connected me to Gene Gollogly at Steiner-Books, and Gene's steady wisdom has been my privilege.

Without Susan Roberson's administrative help, observations, questions, integrity, and good humor, this book would not be.

Brooke Pyeatt, my much-cherished partner, spent his formative years with minimal electricity. His companionship gives me ground.

In the very final days before I turned the book over for final editing, Deb Carney, Larry Glover, Susan Roberson and Char Zehfus each made corrections and contributions that significantly improved it.

And thanks to you, Dear Reader, for joining this roundtable.

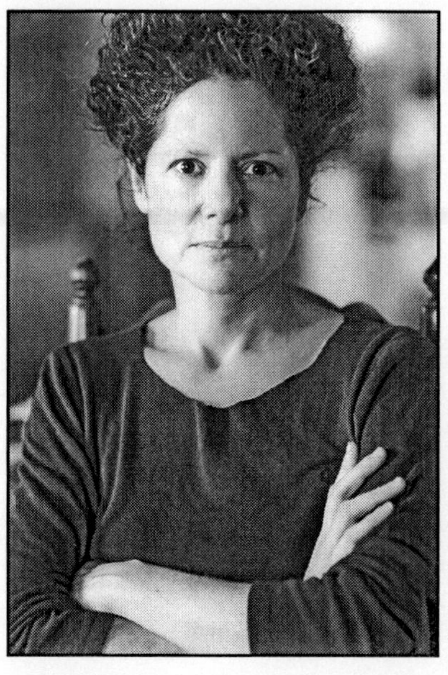

Photo by Jeremy Green

Katie Singer works on public policy with the Electromagnetic Radiation Policy Institute. A medical journalist, her books include *The Garden of Fertility, Honoring Our Cycles* and a novel, *The Wholeness of a Broken Heart*. She teaches internationally. Visit KatieSinger.com, gardenoffertility.com and electronicsilentspring.com.

Lightning Source UK Ltd.
Milton Keynes UK
UKOW04f2348221114

242025UK00002B/54/P